Advance praise for
The Seasonal Kitchen

"There is nothing better than opening Facebook or Instagram and seeing one of Kerry's beautifully displayed, amazing recipes. Not only do they make my mouth water, but they help me to know the fruits and vegetables that are in season and great ways to prepare them. The creativity in preparing and presenting her recipes is often the highlight of my visit to social media!!"

—Randy Farmer-O'Connor, Maryland Public Television, Owings Mills, MD

"Kerry Dunnington combines beautiful flavors and colors so that her dishes not only taste good, but look gorgeous. At the same time, ever conscious of local provender and the changing seasons, Kerry's recipes seem to know just what we're craving."

—Martha Thomas, food editor, *Baltimore Style* magazine, and freelance food writer

"As an avid foodie and home cook, one of my strong beliefs is that 'life happens around the table.' This is how families and friends commiserate and build magical memories, sharing so much and actually talking! Kerry's new cookbook, *The Seasonal Kitchen*, will be one that will make you want to gather everyone around the table, create new traditions, and break bread."

—Ally of Ally's Kitchen, cookbook author, Dole's social media ambassador, and best home cook finalist, Hallmark Channel in 2016

"Kerry Dunnington has managed to incorporate family food traditions with locally sourced products and global ingredients. The result is a must-have cookbook that puts new spins on favorite recipes, like chicken soup (she adds couscous and apricots) and coffee cake (embellished with pineapple cardamom and topped with coconut macadamia streusel). Kerry mentions her mom often in the book, making it a lovely ode to the woman who taught her how to cook."

—Suzanne Loudermilk, restaurant critic, *Baltimore Sun*

"In *The Seasonal Kitchen,* Kerry Dunnington expertly weaves kitchen nostalgia with easy-to-follow culinary instruction and mouthwatering recipes. Each chapter is full of recipes that are perfect not only for today's sophisticated palates, but for all occasions from morning to night as well. Details like the helpful tips and the author's encouragement to view bread making as an art form add extra appeal to *The Seasonal Kitchen*. This volume will inspire newcomers to the kitchen while keeping seasoned cooks satisfied, just as all great cookbooks do!"

—Amy Riolo, award-winning, best-selling author, chef, television personality, cuisine and culture expert, columnist, and Mediterranean diet advocate

"I recently stayed off-season at a friend's condo in Rehoboth Beach, DE. It gave me the opportunity for a little R&R and some downtime to do one of the things I enjoy most—cooking. The well-equipped kitchen in the condo has a very small collection of cookbooks on the counter, and much to my surprise I found one of my all-time favorites, *This Book Cooks,* Kerry Dunnington's highly praised first collection of recipes. I flipped through the pages and was immediately transported into the wonderful, scrumptious world of Kerry's home kitchen.

Well, Kerry is back at it again with an all-new cookbook—*The Seasonal Kitchen*—celebrating real, wholesome food in all its glorious seasons. Kerry has an outstanding palate, and her vast culinary knowledge shines through in her recipe notes and her clear, concise instructions. We are all fortunate to have a new collection of Kerry's vibrant recipes that remind us of the natural world in which we live and the seasonality of food."

—John Shields, author of *Chesapeake Bay Cooking with John Shields*
and chef/owner of Gertrude's Restaurant

"Creating delicious family traditions couldn't be easier with Kerry Dunnington's new cookbook, *The Seasonal Kitchen.* Bring your family back to the dinner table with dishes that will always mean 'home' to those you love."

—Chef Dennis Littley, "A Culinary Journey with Chef Dennis"

"Seasonally eating is a healthy and satisfying ideal, but depending on geography it can be challenging. What does one do with an overabundance of summer squash or a bumper crop of tomatoes? And what to do in the lean winter months? Kerry's recipes offer the solution with unique preparations for everything from spaghetti squash to turnips. *The Seasonal Kitchen* will inspire you to seek out farm-fresh ingredients all year long."

—Christianna McCausland, lifestyle writer

THE SEASONAL KITCHEN

ALSO BY KERRY DUNNINGTON

Tasting the Seasons

This Book Cooks

THE SEASONAL KITCHEN

Farm-Fresh Ingredients Enhance 165 Recipes

KERRY DUNNINGTON

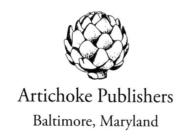

Artichoke Publishers

Baltimore, Maryland

Artichoke Publishers
220 Stoneyford Road
Baltimore, Maryland 21210
www.kerrydunnington.com

Cover photo by Whitney Wasson
Cover and interior design by Anita Jones, Another Jones Graphics
Back cover art and illustrations by Mary "Grace" Bellow-Connor

Publisher's Cataloging-In-Publication Data
(Prepared by The Donohue Group, Inc.)

Names: Dunnington, Kerry. | Bellew-Connor, Mary, illustrator.
Title: The seasonal kitchen : farm-fresh ingredients enhance 165 recipes / Kerry Dunnington ;
    illustrations by Mary "Grace" Bellew-Connor.
Description: Baltimore, Maryland : Artichoke Publishers, [2017] | Includes index.
Identifiers: ISBN 978-0-9904185-6-6
Subjects: LCSH: Seasonal cooking. | Cookery (Natural foods) | Farm produce. | LCGFT: Cookbooks.
Classification: LCC TX714 .D86 2017 | DDC 641.5/64--dc23

Manufactured and printed in the United States of America

DEDICATION

For Nick, the official taste-tester

ACKNOWLEDGMENTS

It takes a team to create a cookbook, and while everyone's role is important, there are some very key players. Nick, my husband of thirty-seven years, is my official taste-tester—the one who always samples each initial recipe and delivers honest and thorough feedback. I am also grateful to family members, friends, neighbors, and longtime catering clients who helped to test the recipes in this book.

Once my recipes were final, I had help in other aspects of compiling the book—editing, proofreading, design, and so forth—and very much appreciate the expertise and input of the following individuals:

Sharon Castlen

Grace Bellew-Connor

Tim Connor

Nick Dunnington

Vince Ercolano

Katherine Gallagher

Anita Jones

Connor Leatherman

Kater Leatherman

Julie Murkette

Robin Reid

Whitney Wasson

About the the artist and illustrator: Mary "Grace" Bellew-Connor is a 17-year-old realism artist who was born in Ho Chi Minh City, Vietnam. She started her art training at the early age of eight, training under the direct supervision of Andy Guerin of the Schuler School of Fine Arts in Baltimore, Maryland. Grace is completing her final year at The Park School of Baltimore and will attend the Tyler School of Art at Temple University in the fall of 2017.

Grace enjoys working in oil while painting her many canine commissions.

CONTENTS

Introducing
THE SEASONAL KITCHEN
xiii–xiv

HAPPY HOUR
Dips
Notable Nibbles
1–20

SOUP DU JOUR
Comfort-Food Soups
Seafood Soups
Vegetarian Soups
21–48

WHAT'S FOR DINNER?
Beef, Lamb, Pork
Chicken and Turkey
Seafood
Vegetarian
49–82

VEGETARIAN SIDE DISHES
Salads
Side Dishes
Potatoes
83–105

BREADS
Rustic Breads
Grain and Seed Breads
Pizza Crust
107–135

EMBELLISHMENTS
Flavored Whipped Cream,
Granola, and Miscellany
137–150

MORNING MEALS
Muffins, Pancakes,
Waffles, and French Toast
Coffee Cakes
Savory Egg Dishes
151–190

THE GRAND FINALE
Cakes, Rolled Cakes,
Pies, Cookies, Ice Cream,
and Dessert Soup
191–231

Product Reference Guide
233–236

Conversion Charts
237–239

Index
241–251

About the Author
253

Introducing
THE SEASONAL KITCHEN

When I was young, the dishes my mother prepared were family-friendly and popular at the time—spaghetti and meatballs, lasagna, meatloaf, pork chops, pot roast, creamed chipped beef, and chicken soup with rivels. Over time, she gained confidence to try new recipes, and through the influence of *The Joy of Cooking*, magazines like *Better Homes and Gardens* and *Family Circle*, and, of course, Julia Child, she began turning out fabulous-tasting gourmet dishes.

Her gourmet ambitions inspired me to begin my own culinary journey. I took an interest in cooking, joining her in the kitchen after school to help prepare dinner. She had few preconceived notions or biases when it came to exploring new culinary possibilities. Together we discovered many unlikely combinations that worked with tasty results. Soon she relinquished Sunday dinner to me.

Initially, I prepared standard fare that was familiar to my sisters and brothers, as well as my parents. Then I began to branch out, elevating my recipes. For example, I added shredded zucchini to my hamburger casserole, topped wedges of iceberg lettuce with homemade blue cheese dressing and crispy garlic croutons, tossed herb butter in with peas and carrots. It wasn't long before I was turning out unlikely and well-seasoned creations of my own. After a few months of cooking and experimenting, I gained confidence and adoration for cooking; my efforts were championed by my parents and siblings.

Shortly after I married, I took the kitchen by storm and set out to re-create more of the tasty home-cooked dishes we'd had growing up. I experimented with many of the excellent recipes my mother had jotted on 5 x 7 index cards and transformed them, adding a variety of pronounced spices, flavor boosters, and rule-bending ingredients. I recorded my creations in a journal that eventually became my first cookbook, *This Book Cooks,* and later my second volume, *Tasting the Seasons.*

Along the way, I have remained loyal to my culinary roots, while creating new combinations and enhancing traditional classics. I encourage my readers to eat fresh fruits and vegetables in season and to support nearby dairy farmers, vendors, and food artisans. When local fruits and vegetables aren't available, I rely on traditionally preserved (tinned or frozen) food—whether mass-produced from companies that adhere to sustainable practices or homemade. I do buy fresh fruits and vegetables that come from different parts of the world when I cannot find them locally; in other words, I rely on global when I can't source local. I'd rather buy what's in season locally or globally than risk buying flavorless strawberries, insipid peaches, or tasteless tomatoes when I can get the most amazing-tasting hand-harvested mangoes from India.

Since my early culinary endeavors, I've been drawn to the magic of cooking and the pleasurable transformation that happens in the kitchen. It's thrilling to transform ingredients into something unexpected and delicious, and in the process, to create next-level versions of standard recipes by combining local and global ingredients. And so I am now overjoyed to be introducing *The Seasonal Kitchen.*

This is a collection of recipes that often combine the local harvest with global foods. I have enlivened and updated these traditional recipes with new and imaginative culinary flair, adding a notable hint of the unexpected to the familiar and balancing treasured traditions with invention and creativity.

For example, in my recipe for chicken soup with couscous and apricots, chicken takes on a whole new meaning. Likewise, summer peaches blend with aromatic cardamom in a coffee cake with almond butter streusel, and my irresistible crispy fritters are made with an unlikely ingredient—spaghetti squash. Then there is the recipe for curry cumin coconut cauliflower finished with sweet prunes and salty peanuts.

In a brunch casserole, I've taken ordinary poached eggs and added them to a combination of fire-roasted tomatoes, garlic, wilted spinach, tender eggplant, Asiago cheese, crispy bacon, and black beans. For a unique salad, garden-harvested arugula is mixed with mango, hearts of palm, coconut, and macadamia nuts and tossed with salty lime dressing. These are a few instances where new culinary accents enliven the dishes I appreciated growing up.

My mission is to give you confidence in the kitchen to make delicious meals. With more than 165 recipes, the book offers ingenious food combinations, enriching stories, innovative and exciting ideas, and recipes that are easy enough for weekday meals and special enough for dinner parties and festive occasions. From morning meals to the grand finale, from sweet to savory, this is a collection of unique, palate-pleasing recipes, including many that are vegetarian.

For my friends across the pond and beyond, I created a conversion chart as well as a valuable product reference guide (page 233) that also includes several useful cooking tips. The introduction page for each chapter includes a lineup of the recipes and a chapter description.

This is a celebration of the joys of pure good food.

From my kitchen to yours,

Giving Thanks

I'm in gratitude to John Forti, Slow Food state governor of Massachusetts, for allowing me to share *Giving Thanks,* an ode to the past, present, and future.

For the earth, air, fire and water;
For the seasons, and the directions of the compass;
For the phases of our lives, and those that came before us;
For those who did not pave the way, but instead, cultivated it;
For those that saved the seeds of a better future,
And acted as stewards of our resources and inheritance,
A legacy of waterways, woodlands, fields and farms.
An inheritance of seasonal observations, life skills,
holiday customs, recipes for nourishing foods,
deep connections and life passages that anchor us in a sense of place,
stewardship and community.
A celebration in what we have learned thus far, and where we are going.
So I offer this humble prayer to the Native and the immigrant.
For the seacoast and the soil, the seeds and roots,
and the farmers who renew tradition with each passing season.
For the farmers market and the holiday table, our family and friends,
and the kinship that comes from celebrating renewal for our changing landscape and nature!

www.jforti.com

Happy Hour

DIPS AND NOTABLE NIBBLES

The start of the evening—the transition period from day to night—is ideal for mingling with family and friends. You will want the menu to be very special. Here is a collection of our favorite hors d'oeuvres. Many are a rendition of an appetizer my mother served when she was entertaining. Like her, I love serving dips. They tend to be the ideal party dish because they can be made ahead, are most flavorful at room temperature, and are easy to eat by hand. The notable nibbles are more elaborate, sturdier foods (sometimes requiring a small plate and fork) suited for cocktail parties or hearty eaters. Once you've explored the recipes in this chapter, you'll have an irresistible selection of crowd-pleasing party food.

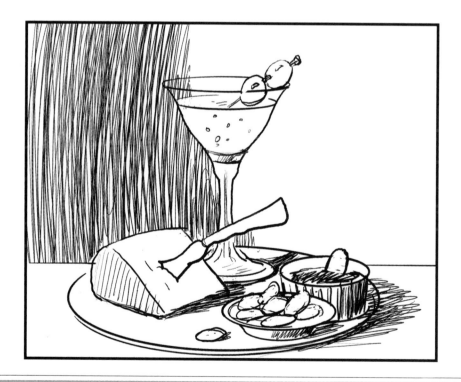

RECIPE INDEX

DIPS

Herb-Infused Bean Dip 3

Creamy Horseradish and Chili Sauce Dip with Shrimp 4

Roasted Red Pepper Hummus Dip with Layered Vegetables, Feta, and Olives 5

Vegetarian Mediterranean Dip 6

Three-Cheese and Roasted Vegetable Dip 7

Creamy Onion and Red Pepper Cheese Dip 8

Hot Cheddar and Cauliflower Dip 9

Cheesy Broccoli and Mushroom Dip 10

NOTABLE NIBBLES

Lemon Rosemary Chicken Wings 11

Coconut Curried Cheese with Mango Chutney 12

Puff Pastry with Creamy Mushroom Filling 13-14

French-Dressed Apricot Chicken Wings 15

New England-Like Lobster Pies 16

Spinach Parmesan Bites 17

Colman's Deviled Eggs with Tarragon 18

Three-Cheese Spaghetti Squash Fritters 19-20

HERB-INFUSED BEAN DIP

This quick, easy, make-ahead appetizer recipe uses a lot of fresh parsley that turns this nutrient-rich dip a beautiful shade of green. It also uses Spike, a salt-free seasoning made from thirty-nine exotic herbs, spices, and vegetables. Serve the dip with crostini, tortilla chips, or sturdy fresh vegetables. Spike's line of seasonings can be found in the spice aisle of most health-oriented grocery stores nationwide or online.

About 8 servings

1 can (15 ounces) white beans (cannellini, navy, great northern), drained
½ cup onion, cut into chunks
1 cup loosely packed fresh parsley
2 tablespoons lemon juice
2 cloves garlic
2 teaspoons Spike
1 teaspoon salt
Several grindings of black pepper
Fresh snipped chives (garnish)

1. In a food processor, pulse the beans with the onion. Add parsley, lemon juice, garlic, Spike, salt, and black pepper. Process until the mixture is smooth and creamy.
2. Serve immediately or cover and refrigerate until serving time. Just before serving, garnish the dip with snipped chives.

CREAMY HORSERADISH AND CHILI SAUCE DIP WITH SHRIMP

Soon after my mother moved from the home she had lived in for twenty-nine years to a retirement home, we spent many afternoons in her new place going through her vast collection of recipes. This recipe for shrimp dip, written in her beautiful script, was marked with four stars next to the title—her code for excellent. She first tasted it at a neighborhood cocktail party. It was a hit then, and was a hit when I took it to a potluck party. Serve with either a neutral-flavored cracker, bagel chips, or pita chips. If you're not familiar with it, chili sauce is a condiment made with chili peppers and tomatoes. This dip is best made in advance. For my favorite brand of horseradish, see the Product Reference Guide on page 233.

10 to 12 servings

One package (8 ounces, block-style) ⅓ less fat cream cheese, at room temperature
½ cup mayonnaise
½ cup chili sauce
½ cup sweet onion, finely chopped
2 teaspoons prepared horseradish
1 cup cooked shrimp, chopped
Fresh snipped chives (garnish)

1. In a medium bowl, combine the cream cheese, mayonnaise, chili sauce, onion, and horseradish. Blend until fully combined. Add the shrimp and stir until incorporated.
2. Transfer the mixture to a rimmed serving dish. Cover and refrigerate for several hours. Just before serving, garnish the dip with chives.

ROASTED RED PEPPER HUMMUS DIP WITH LAYERED VEGETABLES, FETA, AND OLIVES

This healthy, colorful, and tasty dip is one of my go-to dips when I need to make an appetizer in advance. Pita chips are a complementing accompaniment.

8 servings

1 container (8 ounces) roasted red pepper hummus
1 cup plain Greek-style yogurt
1 jar (6 ounces) marinated artichoke hearts, drained, roughly chopped
1 cup cucumbers, peeled, seeded, and diced
⅓ cup sun-dried tomatoes, drained of any liquid and chopped
⅓ cup Kalamata olives, pitted and chopped
¼ cup thinly sliced scallions (green onion)
⅓ cup feta cheese, crumbled

1. Spread the hummus evenly in the bottom of an 8-inch rimmed dish. Spread the yogurt evenly over the hummus. Scatter the artichokes over the yogurt. Scatter the cucumbers, sun-dried tomatoes, and olives over the artichoke hearts. Top the artichoke hearts with the scallions and feta cheese. Serve immediately or cover and refrigerate until serving time.

VEGETARIAN MEDITERRANEAN DIP

This is very similar to the popular recipe for hummus dip with layered vegetables, feta, and olives (page 5). Here I've added healthy spinach and roasted red peppers with tasty results. If you're pressed for time, this colorful dip can be made in advance. Serve with pita chips.

8 servings

1 container (8 ounces) hummus
1 cup plain Greek-style yogurt
1 jar (6 ounces) marinated artichoke hearts, drained, roughly chopped
10 ounces chopped cooked spinach, squeezed dry
½ cup roasted red peppers, drained, roughly chopped
⅓ cup Kalamata olives, pitted and chopped
¼ cup thinly sliced scallions (green onions)
⅓ cup feta cheese, crumbled

1. Spread the hummus evenly in the bottom of an 8-inch rimmed dish. Spread the yogurt evenly over the hummus. Scatter the artichoke hearts over the yogurt. Scatter the spinach, peppers, and olives over the artichoke hearts. Top the artichoke hearts with the scallions and feta cheese. Serve immediately or cover and refrigerate until serving time.

THREE-CHEESE AND ROASTED VEGETABLE DIP

I love to roast a medley of vegetables and keep them on hand. Roasting is simple. For directions, see the Product Reference Guide (page 233). This recipe received rave reviews at a potluck party. Accompany with a neutral cracker or crostini.

About 8 to 10 servings

1 cup assorted roasted vegetables
½ cup crumbled feta cheese
½ cup freshly shredded cheddar cheese
½ cup freshly grated Parmesan cheese
1 cup mayonnaise

1. Preheat the oven to 350°F.
2. In a medium bowl, combine the roasted vegetables with the feta, cheddar, Parmesan, and mayonnaise.
3. Transfer the mixture to a 1-quart baking dish. Bake for 30 to 45 minutes or until light brown and bubbly. Serve immediately.

CREAMY ONION AND RED PEPPER CHEESE DIP

Fair warning: This creamy, cheesy, chock-full-of-onion-flavor dip is a crowd-pleaser that tasters tend to hover over. Serve it with a thin, crispy cracker—rye and pumpernickel are especially complementing.

Serves a crowd

1 cup leeks, thinly sliced
1 cup Vidalia onion, chopped
1 cup white onion, chopped
3 packages (8 ounces each, block-style) ⅓ less fat cream cheese, at room temperature
1¼ cups freshly grated Parmesan cheese
1 cup mayonnaise
2 large cloves garlic, minced
1½ teaspoons salt
½ teaspoon red pepper flakes
Fresh ground black pepper to taste
Fresh snipped chives (garnish)

1. In a medium pot over moderate heat, bring ½ cup of water to a boil. Add the leeks, Vidalia onion, and white onion. Bring the mixture to a boil, reduce the heat to simmer, and cook for about 15 minutes or until the onions are tender. Drain the liquid from the onions. (Liquid can be saved and used as a base for soup broth.)
2. Preheat the oven to 400°F.
3. In a large bowl, combine the cream cheese with one cup of the Parmesan cheese, mayonnaise, garlic, salt, red pepper flakes, and pepper. Add the onions and combine until well blended.
4. Transfer the mixture to an 8-inch baking dish. Top the mixture with the remaining ¼ cup of Parmesan cheese. Bake for 30 minutes or until light brown and bubbly. Garnish the dip with chives. Serve immediately.

HOT CHEDDAR AND CAULIFLOWER DIP

This is a creamy, cheesy, comforting appetizer to serve when the air is crisp, the temperatures have fallen, and you're ready to cozy up in front of a roaring fire. Serve with pita chips or crostini.

8 to 10 servings

2½ cups cauliflower florets
4 ounces (block-style) ⅓ less fat cream cheese, at room temperature
¼ cup mayonnaise
2 cloves garlic, minced
¾ teaspoon salt
½ teaspoon red pepper flakes
3½ cups shredded sharp cheddar cheese

1. Preheat the oven to 350°F.
2. In a medium pot fitted with a steamer, cook the cauliflower until fork-tender. Immediately remove the florets from the steamer pot. When the cauliflower is cool enough to handle, break into bite-sized pieces and place in a medium bowl.
3. In a small bowl, combine the cream cheese, mayonnaise, garlic, salt, red pepper flakes, and cheese until well blended.
4. Transfer the mixture to a 9-inch baking dish and bake for about 30 minutes or until lightly brown and bubbly. Serve immediately.

CHEESY BROCCOLI AND MUSHROOM DIP

Your party guests will devour this irresistible dip. Accompany with pita chips or crostini. If you're desirous of a spicy version, use a hot pepper cheddar cheese, like habanero.

8 to 10 servings

2 cups broccoli florets
1 tablespoon butter
1 cup sweet onion, finely chopped
1 package (4 ounces) or about 1½ cups baby shitake mushrooms, finely chopped
¾ teaspoon salt
A few grindings of black pepper
¼ cup white wine
2 cups shredded sharp cheddar cheese
½ cup sour cream
4 ounces (block-style) ⅓ less fat cream cheese, at room temperature

1. In a medium pot fitted with a steamer, cook the broccoli until fork-tender, about 5 to 7 minutes. Immediately remove the florets from the pot. When the broccoli is cool enough to handle, break into bite-sized pieces and place in a medium bowl.
2. Preheat the oven to 350°F.
3. Generously oil an 8-inch baking dish with cooking spray.
4. In a medium skillet, melt the butter over medium-high heat. Add the onion and cook, stirring often, until slightly browned, about 5 minutes. Add the mushrooms, salt, and pepper, and cook until the mushrooms are tender. Add the wine and cook for about 2 minutes. Remove the skillet from the heat.
5. Add the broccoli to the onion/mushroom mixture and stir to combine.
6. In a medium bowl, combine the cheddar cheese, sour cream, and cream cheese. Stir until well blended. Add the broccoli/mushroom mixture to the cheese mixture and combine until well distributed. Don't worry about the broccoli breaking up when combining with the cheese mixture.
7. Transfer the mixture to the prepared baking dish. Bake for about 30 minutes or until bubbly. Serve immediately.

LEMON ROSEMARY CHICKEN WINGS

Every year we kick off summer and commemorate Memorial Day with family and friends. The menu varies from year to year, but I often serve these wings because of their popularity. Plan accordingly; the wings need to marinate at least eight hours or overnight.

About 24 chicken wings

4 pounds chicken wings
½ cup olive oil
½ cup lemon juice
⅓ cup rosemary leaves
5 cloves garlic, minced, about 2 tablespoons
1 teaspoon coarse salt
Several grindings of black pepper
Rosemary sprigs and lemons wedges (garnish)

1. Place the chicken wings in a large rimmed dish.
2. In a medium bowl, combine the olive oil, lemon juice, rosemary leaves, garlic, salt, and pepper. Whisk until well combined. Pour the marinade over the wings. Cover and refrigerate. Marinate for 8 hours or overnight, turning the wings once or twice.
3. Preheat the oven to 400°F.
4. Line a large rimmed baking sheet with parchment paper.
5. Transfer the wings and marinade to the baking sheet, and arrange in a single layer. Bake the wings uncovered for about 15 minutes. Turn and bake an additional 15 minutes or until cooked through and golden brown. Transfer the wings to a serving platter and garnish the platter with rosemary sprigs and lemon wedges. Serve immediately.

COCONUT CURRIED CHEESE WITH MANGO CHUTNEY

Serve this vibrant-tasting, palate-pleasing appetizer with raisin crostini. The cheese-to-chutney ratio is a matter of preference. I use about a half cup, then add more if needed.

About 10 to 15 servings

One package (8 ounces, block-style) ⅓ less fat cream cheese, at room temperature
1 cup shredded sharp white cheddar cheese
2 tablespoons cooking sherry
1 teaspoon curry powder
¼ cup chopped dried apricots
¼ cup shredded sweetened coconut (plus extra for garnish)
¼ cup chopped pecans (plus extra for garnish)
Mango chutney, about ½ to 1 cup

1. In a medium bowl, combine the cream cheese, cheddar cheese, sherry, curry powder, apricots, coconut, and pecans. Mix until thoroughly combined.
2. Transfer the mixture to a rimmed serving dish and form into a flat round shape, about 6 inches in diameter. Using a soup ladle, make an indentation in the center of the round.
3. If you're serving immediately, cover the top of the cheese with the mango chutney. Top the chutney with the extra shredded coconut and chopped pecans. If you're not serving immediately, cover the cheese and refrigerate until serving time. Just prior to serving, top the cheese with the chutney and the shredded coconut and chopped pecans. Serve immediately.

PUFF PASTRY WITH CREAMY MUSHROOM FILLING

These crispy, creamy morsels are very well received, and they're great to serve for a special celebration, especially if you're hosting a large crowd, because the yield is large. Take note: The mushroom filling must be prepared the day before you fill the puff pastry. Puff pastry needs to thaw before it's ready to roll. Not every brand has the same thawing instructions; check the directions before you begin to roll the pastry. You can be creative with the selection of mushrooms; a variety is fun, and, of course, shitake mushrooms are so flavorful.

80 pieces–about 20 per roll

4 tablespoons butter
1 package (10 ounces or about 13 to 15 medium-sized) white mushrooms,
 finely chopped
3 tablespoons unbleached all-purpose flour
1 cup heavy cream
1 teaspoon salt
½ teaspoon onion powder
1 tablespoon cooking sherry
2 boxes puff pastry sheets, thawed according to package directions
1 egg, lightly beaten

1. In a medium skillet over moderate heat, melt the butter and sauté the mushrooms for about 5 minutes. Whisk in the flour, 1 tablespoon at a time. Slowly whisk in the heavy cream and stir until the cream is combined with the mushrooms. Add the salt, onion powder, and sherry. Cook until the mixture thickens. Remove the skillet from the heat and allow the mixture to cool. Transfer to a container, cover, and refrigerate overnight.
2. Line 2 rimmed baking sheets with parchment paper.
3. Unfold the pastry sheets onto a lightly floured surface. Working with one pastry sheet at a time, gently roll each pastry sheet to remove the fold marks. Using a knife or spatula, divide the mushroom filling into four equal parts—this will give you the approximate amount to use for each pastry sheet.
4. Spread the mushroom filling evenly over each puff pastry sheet, leaving a ½-inch border.

Starting with the short side, roll the pastry jelly roll fashion. Place the stuffed puff pastry roll seam side down on the prepared baking sheet. Refrigerate the rolls for 15 minutes or until the puff pastry is firm.

5. Preheat the oven to 375°F.

6. Cut each roll into ½-inch slices. Place the slices cut side down on the prepared baking sheets. Brush each slice with beaten egg. Bake for 15 to 20 minutes or until golden. Allow the slices to cool for several minutes before serving.

FRENCH-DRESSED APRICOT CHICKEN WINGS

People devour these chicken wings! We like our wings with lots of sauce. If you would rather they not be swimming in sauce, add the desired amount of sauce and use the rest as a topping for meatloaf or your next batch of apricot chicken wings. I use Annie's French dressing because I like the authentic taste. I also like the company's philosophy. Simply Organic makes a wonderful French onion dip mix. For a lovely presentation, serve the wings on a bed of shredded savoy cabbage.

About 24 chicken wings

1 bottle (8 ounces) French dressing
1 cup apricot preserves
1 package (1.10 ounce) onion dip mix
1 tablespoon dried minced onion
4 pounds chicken wings
Freshly shredded savoy cabbage (garnish)

1. Preheat the oven to 400°F.
2. Line a rimmed baking sheet with parchment paper.
3. In a large bowl, combine the French dressing, apricot preserves, onion dip mix, and minced onion. Add the wings and toss with the sauce to coat the wings evenly. Transfer the wings to the prepared baking sheet.
4. Bake for 15 minutes. Turn the wings over and bake an additional 15 minutes. Switch the oven temperature to broil and broil the wings on each side until slightly blackened. Allow the wings to cool slightly before transferring to a platter. Arrange the wings on a bed of shredded savoy cabbage.

NEW ENGLAND-LIKE LOBSTER PIES

I often serve these elegant bite-sized morsels at catered parties. They fly off the servers' trays, and for obvious reasons. The combination is reminiscent of the popular New England lobster roll, hence their name. Here, instead of heaps of creamy lobster between toasted, buttered bread, this tasty mixture goes into those ever-so-popular crispy mini phyllo shells.

About 60 miniature pies

2 pounds lobster meat, cooked and chopped into bite-sized pieces
½ cup onion, finely chopped
½ cup celery, finely chopped
½ cup green or red pepper, finely chopped
1 cup mayonnaise
½ teaspoon salt
1 teaspoon Worcestershire sauce
⅛ teaspoon cracked black pepper
4 boxes (15 count each) mini phyllo shells (aka filo and fillo)

1. Preheat the oven to 350°F.
2. Lined a rimmed baking sheet with parchment paper.
3. In a large bowl, combine the onion, celery, pepper, mayonnaise, salt, Worcestershire sauce, and black pepper. Fold the lobster into the mayonnaise mixture, and mix until well combined.
4. Fill the shells and bake for 5 to 10 minutes or until heated through. Or cover and refrigerate until you're ready to fill the shells. (It's important to fill the shells just prior to baking; otherwise the shells will get soggy.) Serve immediately.

SPINACH PARMESAN BITES

Serve these cheesy spinach bites on their own or with your favorite marinara sauce for dipping.

6 servings, 3 per person

¼ cup butter
½ cup finely chopped onion
2 cloves garlic, minced
2 eggs
16 ounces frozen chopped spinach, defrosted, drained, and squeezed dry
1 cup herb-seasoned stuffing
1 cup freshly grated Parmesan cheese
A few grindings of black pepper
¼ teaspoon nutmeg

1. Preheat the oven to 350°F.
2. In a medium sauté pan, melt the butter over moderate heat and sauté the onion until transparent. Add the garlic and sauté for about 2 minutes.
3. In a large bowl, beat the eggs and add the spinach, stuffing, Parmesan cheese, black pepper, and nutmeg. Mix until the ingredients are fully incorporated.
4. Shape the mixture into bite-sized balls—about 18 pieces. Place the balls on a rimmed, parchment-lined baking sheet. Bake for 15 to 20 minutes, or until light golden brown on the bottom. Serve warm.

COLMAN'S DEVILED EGGS WITH TARRAGON

The distinctive flavor that makes this deviled egg recipe so delicious is the Colman's mustard and tarragon vinegar. To get the full flavor of the mustard, it's important that the mustard be mixed with the cold water and allowed to stand for 10 minutes. The water acts as a catalyst that helps yield the essential oil of the mustard, which produces the unmistakable taste. Eggs vary in size, so season with more vinegar, Worcestershire sauce, and mayonnaise until the flavors hit that just perfect comfort-food note. Colman's mustard can be found in the spice aisle of most grocery stores nationwide. For an eye-catching presentation, I like to place the eggs on a bed of sweet pea shoots, shredded carrots, or thinly sliced watermelon radishes. Microgreens add a lovely contrast of color as a garnish on top of the eggs.

Serves 6

1 dozen large eggs, hard-boiled, peeled
1 teaspoon Colman's mustard
1 teaspoon cold water
Salt and pepper to taste
¼ cup fresh minced parsley
1 teaspoon tarragon vinegar, or more to taste
½ teaspoon Worcestershire sauce, or more to taste
½ cup mayonnaise or more to make a creamy mixture
Microgreens (garnish)

1. In a small bowl, mix the Colman's mustard with the cold water. Let the mixture stand for 10 minutes.
2. Cut the eggs in half and transfer the yolks to a medium bowl. Mash the yolks with a fork. Season the yolks with salt and pepper. Add the parsley and stir to combine.
3. In a small bowl, combine the vinegar, Worcestershire sauce, mustard, and mayonnaise. Fold into the egg yolk mixture and mix until well blended. Adjust seasonings and add additional vinegar, Worcestershire sauce, and mayonnaise if necessary.
4. Fill the egg white halves with the yolk mixture. Cover and refrigerate until serving time or serve immediately. Garnish with microgreens if desired.

THREE-CHEESE SPAGHETTI SQUASH FRITTERS

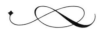

More often than not, tasters don't detect the spaghetti squash and comment how much they love the *cheese fritters*! I like the fritters' ragged appearance, so don't worry about forming them. Just pull off small amounts of batter and drop them into the hot oil. Plan accordingly; fritter batter is best made a day in advance. Also, the spaghetti squash must be cooked before adding it to the batter. Directions for how to prepare and cook spaghetti squash can be found in the Product Reference Guide (page 233). Just about any flavorful and good melting cheese works in this recipe. These fritters are delicious on their own, but if you want to serve them with an accompanying sauce, roasted eggplant tomato sauce is a favorite. For a lively flavor, serve them with harissa. For the recipe, see poached eggs over couscous with a pop of harissa heat on page 187.

If you don't have a thermometer to check the temperature of the oil, you can test it by adding a kernel of popcorn; if it pops immediately, the oil is hot enough to fry. A grain of white rice also works to test the temperature. If it pops right back to the top and starts cooking, the oil is ready for frying. Golden-colored fritters are beautiful when served on a bed of savoy cabbage leaves.

About 16 to 20 fritters (depending on desired size)

1½ cups unbleached all-purpose flour
2 teaspoons baking powder
½ teaspoon salt
2 cups chopped spaghetti squash
½ cup grated fontina cheese
½ cup freshly grated Parmesan
1 cup shredded mozzarella cheese
1 tablespoon minced onion
1 egg
1 cup milk
High-heat oil for frying (avocado, peanut, or sunflower oil)
Savoy cabbage leaves for platter

1. In a large bowl, combine the flour, baking powder, and salt. Add the chopped spaghetti squash, cheese, and onion, and stir until fully combined.

2. In a small bowl, whisk together the egg and milk. Add to the flour mixture and stir just to combine. Cover and refrigerate overnight.

3. In a large pot, heat 4 to 6 inches of oil over moderately high heat.

4. When the oil is hot, drop small amounts of the fritter batter into the oil (the fritters expand after they're dropped into the hot oil) and cook them, turning once or twice until they are golden brown. Using a slotted spoon, transfer the fritters to a paper towel-lined platter.

5. Allow the fritters to cool slightly before transferring them to a serving platter. Serve immediately.

Soup du Jour

COMFORT-FOOD SOUPS
SEAFOOD SOUPS
VEGETARIAN SOUPS

Gathered here is an assortment of taste-testers' favorite soups that have pleased many palates. When I was developing recipes for this book, I became increasingly bold in my creations. After I discovered the amazing flavor that came from combining ginger, coconut, and mellow-tasting vegetables, I created several soups using that winning combination. There are many innovative combinations in this chapter, including recipes for curried pumpkin soup with mushrooms, gingered butternut squash soup with coconut, chicken soup with couscous and apricots, and coconut black bean soup with mango and avocado salsa. Whether you're hosting lunch or dinner, a seated dinner party or a casual luncheon, you will find something that perfectly suits the particular appetites—vegetarian, vegan, or hearty carnivore—of those at your table.

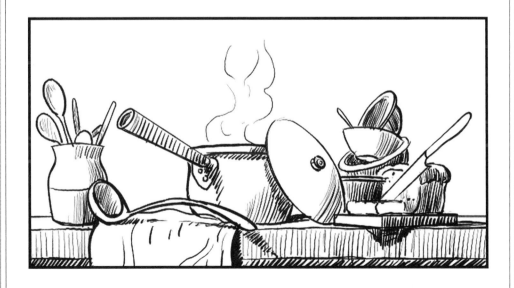

My mother frowned upon food waste. Although we were encouraged to finish everything put in front of us, she was more concerned about minimizing waste during preparation. The water left over from steaming vegetables or boiling potatoes and noodles, the essence from cooked chicken or beef—these she saved as the foundation for that next pot of wonderful soup. I adopted this way of collecting flavored liquids and essence and often use them as the basis for my soup stocks.

I realize that in today's busy and fast-moving kitchens, not every cook has the inclination to do this. Hence, many of the soup recipes in this chapter call for a vegetable bouillon cube. After taste-testing various brands, I found Rapunzel was the one bursting with abundant flavor. My go-to brand for chicken broth is Imagine Organic Chicken Broth; like Rapunzel, it has a rich flavor that's close to homemade. Muir Glen is my favored tomato brand. When fresh vegetables aren't in season, I rely on traditionally preserved food, whether tinned or frozen; for example, tinned beans and frozen peas, spinach, corn, and green beans are recommended if fresh ones are not readily available.

RECIPE INDEX

COMFORT-FOOD SOUPS

Cauliflower Soup with Cheddar Ciabatta Toast 24

Creamy Fire-Roasted Tomato Soup 25

Potato and Corn Chowder with Bacon 26

Creamy Coconut and Cauliflower Soup with Tandoori Spice 27

Chicken Soup with Couscous and Apricots 28

Ham and White Bean Soup 29

Savory-Sweet Parsnip and Sweet Potato Soup 30

SEAFOOD SOUPS

Fire-Roasted Seafood-Style Chili 31

Creamy Lobster Soup 32

Shrimp and Coconut Soup with Roasted Corn and Sweet Potato 33-34

Cucumber and Crab Soup 35

VEGETARIAN SOUPS

Curried Pumpkin Soup with Mushrooms 36

Gingered Butternut Squash Soup with Coconut 37

Creamy Wild Mushroom Soup with Turmeric 38

Vegetable Chowder with Cheese Tortellini 39

Cream of Turnip Soup with Pumpernickel Croutons 40

Coconut Black Bean Soup with Mango and Avocado Salsa 41-42

Mushroom Soup with Spinach Tortellini 43

Gingered Turnip Soup with Coconut 44

Green Bean Casserole Soup 45-46

Gingered Coconut and Celery Soup 47

Winter Solstice Soup 48

Cauliflower Soup with Cheddar Ciabatta Toast

When this mild-tasting vegetable comes into season, I love to make this creamy, soothing soup. The crispy, cheesy toast adds a wonderful contrast of textures. For a pop of beautiful color, use either purple or golden-yellow cauliflower instead of white.

6 servings

2 tablespoons butter
1 cup sliced onion
2 cups chicken broth
1½ pounds cauliflower, broken into uniform pieces
1 vegetable bouillon cube
1 teaspoon salt
2 tablespoons cooking sherry
Several grindings of black pepper
6 slices ciabatta bread
Shredded sharp cheddar cheese
Fresh snipped chives (garnish)

1. Melt the butter in a large pot over moderate heat. Add the onion and sauté until translucent. Add the chicken broth, cauliflower, and bouillon cube. Cover and bring the mixture to a boil, reduce the heat to simmer, and cook until cauliflower is fork-tender, about 20 minutes. Add the salt, sherry, and black pepper.
2. In a food processor or blender, purée the soup in batches, and transfer the puréed batches into a large bowl. After the final batch is puréed, transfer the soup back into the original large pot, and simmer until ready to serve.
3. Set the oven temperature to broil.
4. Line a rimmed baking sheet with parchment paper. Arrange the slices of bread in a single layer and top with shredded cheddar cheese. Place under the broiler and broil until the cheese has melted and is lightly brown in spots. Watch closely so as not to burn the cheese toast.
5. Ladle soup into 6 serving bowls and partially nestle each bowl with cheddar ciabatta toast. Garnish with chives if desired. Serve immediately.

CREAMY FIRE-ROASTED TOMATO SOUP

The tomato soup and grilled cheese sandwich combo is an American comfort food like no other. Just the thought of the duo takes me back to my grandparents' home where I recall, with pure joy, savoring steaming bowls of smooth-as-cream tomato soup with crispy, chestnut-colored, buttery sandwiches oozing with drippy cheese. In one word: Amazeballs. Here, instead of using traditionally preserved tomatoes, I've added Muir Glen's brand of organic fire-roasted tomatoes for an authentic, robust tomato flavor that takes this traditional favorite to the next level. My preferred brand for store-bought chicken broth, for its full-bodied flavor, is Imagine.

8 servings

*3 tablespoons neutral oil (expeller-pressed canola, high-oleic safflower, or
  sunflower oil)*
3 cups chopped sweet onion
3 cloves garlic, minced
4 cups chicken broth
1 can (28 ounces) fire-roasted tomatoes
1 teaspoon salt
Several grindings of black pepper
½ cup heavy cream

1. Heat the oil in a large pot over moderate heat. Add the onions and cook for 10 to 15 minutes, stirring occasionally, until golden brown. Add the garlic and cook for 1 minute. Add the chicken broth, tomatoes, salt, and pepper. Bring the mixture to a boil, reduce the heat, and simmer for about 15 minutes.
2. In a food processor or blender, purée the soup in batches and transfer the puréed batches into a large bowl. Transfer all the puréed soup back into the original large pot, add the cream, and stir to blend. Simmer until heated through. Serve immediately.

POTATO AND CORN CHOWDER WITH BACON

Potatoes, summer corn from the cob, butter, cream, and bacon? Faithful food aficionados, don your aprons and start cooking! For a contrast of textures, I like to chop two cups of the corn and keep the remaining two cups of kernels whole.

8 servings

6 tablespoons butter
3 cups onion, chopped
1 cup celery, chopped
3 cups potatoes, cubed
1 container (32-ounce) chicken broth
4 cups fresh corn kernels
2 cups cream
⅓ cup sherry
2 teaspoons salt
Several grindings of black pepper
6 slices of bacon, cooked and crumbled
Fresh snipped chives (garnish)

1. Melt the butter in a large pot over medium heat, and sauté the onion and celery for about 3 minutes. Add the potatoes and the chicken broth and bring the mixture to a boil. Cover, reduce the heat to medium, and cook until the potatoes are tender, about 10 minutes.
2. Roughly chop 2 cups of the corn and add them to the soup. Add the remaining corn and cream, and season with salt and pepper. Blend until fully incorporated. Add the bacon and simmer until ready to serve.

CREAMY COCONUT AND CAULIFLOWER SOUP WITH TANDOORI SPICE

This is a mouthful in more ways than one. It has such an interesting group of local and global ingredients with so many colors, textures, and flavors—and it's one of our favorites. The bounty of ingredients turns this delicious soup the most gorgeous shade of pumpkin. It's perfect to serve on a cold winter's night in front of a roaring fire. Taste-testers' favorite pairing is cast-iron honey-glazed cornbread (page 115).

8 to 10 servings

⅓ cup uncooked wild rice
1 tablespoon coconut oil
1 medium sweet potato, peeled and cubed
1 cup chopped onion
1 cup chopped celery
2 cups cauliflower, broken into bite-sized pieces
1 tablespoon tandoori spice blend
2 cups chicken broth
1 can (14.5 ounces) fire-roasted tomatoes
1 can (14 ounces) coconut milk
1 can (14 ounces) white beans
2 vegetable bouillon cubes
½ cup chunky natural peanut butter

1. Cook the wild rice according to the package directions. While the rice is cooking, prepare the soup.
2. In a large pot, heat the oil over moderate heat and sauté the sweet potato, onion, celery, and cauliflower for about 5 minutes. Add the tandoori spice blend and sauté for about 1 minute. Add the chicken broth. Cover the pot and bring the mixture to a boil, reduce the heat to medium, and cook for 10 to 15 minutes or until the vegetables are tender.
3. Add the tomatoes, coconut milk, beans, bouillon cubes, and peanut butter. Stir until the cubes have dissolved and the peanut butter and coconut milk are evenly distributed. Reduce the heat to a simmer. When the rice has finished cooking, add it to the soup and stir until well combined. Serve immediately.

CHICKEN SOUP WITH COUSCOUS AND APRICOTS

Recipe development is all about textures and contrasts and building a balanced bite. The apricots and prunes are a stunning complement to the chicken, vegetables, and couscous. Plan accordingly; the chicken is cooked before it is added to the soup. For my favorite chicken broth brand, see the Product Reference Guide, page 233.

4 servings

½ cup plain uncooked couscous
1 tablespoon neutral oil (expeller-pressed canola, high-oleic safflower, or sunflower oil)
1 cup thinly sliced leeks
1½ cups sliced celery
8 cups chicken broth
1 cup green beans, fresh or frozen
2 cups cooked white-meat chicken, torn into bite-sized pieces
½ cup chopped dried apricots
½ cup chopped pitted prunes
1 cup fresh cilantro leaves, chopped
1 tablespoon dark sesame oil
1 tablespoon tamari or soy sauce
Several grindings of black pepper

1. Cook the couscous according to the package directions. Set aside.
2. In a large pot over moderate heat, heat the oil and sauté the leeks and celery for about 5 minutes. Add the chicken broth and green beans and bring the mixture to a boil. Reduce the heat and cook for about 5 minutes or until the vegetables are fork-tender.
3. Add the apricots, prunes, chicken, cilantro, sesame oil, tamari, pepper, and couscous to the mixture. Cook until heated through. Serve immediately.

HAM AND WHITE BEAN SOUP

Growing up, we ate bowls of hearty ham and bean soup (ham from my mother's family-famous recipe in *This Book Cooks*) on many cold winter nights, and it satisfied in the most complete way. If you don't have leftover ham, ask the butcher for a slab or get a thick slice from the deli section. We always accompany this soup with cornbread—the recipe for cast-iron honey-glazed cornbread on page 115 is very complementing.

4 to 6 servings

2 cups water
1 cup carrots, julienned
1 cup celery, chopped
1 cup onion, chopped
¼ cup parsley, chopped
1 vegetable bouillon cube
2 cans (15 ounces each) white beans, (cannellini, navy, great northern)
4 ounces chopped ham
1 tablespoon cooking sherry
A few grindings of black pepper

1. In a medium pot, bring the water to a boil. Add the carrots, celery, onion, and parsley. Reduce the heat slightly and cook until the vegetables are tender, about 10 minutes.
2. Add the bouillon cube and stir until it is dissolved. Add the beans and ham. Season with sherry and black pepper. Simmer the soup until ready to serve.

Savory-Sweet Parsnip and Sweet Potato Soup

Parsnips are lamentably underappreciated, but they are one of the tastiest winter vegetables, so sweet and deep-flavored. Parsnips' sweetness is enhanced by cold temperatures, and that's when I prepare this soothing, creamy soup. You'll want to pass over enormous parsnips. They tend to be woody and tough—not sweet and tender, like the small-to-medium-sized parsnips. If you're not a fan of this sweet root vegetable, consider giving this recipe a try. It might completely change your opinion about parsnips.

8 servings

2 tablespoons butter
1 cup onion, chopped
1 cup celery, chopped
1 teaspoon cinnamon
¼ teaspoon nutmeg
4 cups chicken broth
1 pound parsnips, peeled and cut into uniform chunks
2 pounds sweet potatoes, peeled and cubed
1 teaspoon salt
1½ cups milk

1. In a large pot, melt the butter over medium heat. Sauté the onion and celery until tender. Add the cinnamon and nutmeg and sauté until fragrant, about 1 minute. Add the chicken broth, parsnips, and sweet potatoes. Bring the mixture to a boil. Cover, lower the heat, and cook until the parsnips and sweet potatoes are tender, about 30 to 40 minutes.

2. Purée the mixture in a food processor or blender in batches, and then transfer the mixture into a large bowl as it's puréed. Add the salt and milk to the last batch to be puréed and transfer back into the original large pot. Simmer until heated through. Serve immediately.

FIRE-ROASTED SEAFOOD-STYLE CHILI

Fire-roasted tomatoes add a rich, smoky flavor to this robust version of traditional chili made with ground beef. This is a wonderful departure from conventional chili. Here the beans and seafood crowd a highly seasoned tomato broth. Serve with cast-iron honey-glazed cornbread (page 115) and a tossed lettuce leaf salad for a completely satisfying, elegant meal your guests won't soon forget. It's best to prepare this a day in advance to allow the intense flavors to mingle. If the amount of chili seasoning seems too aggressive, start by using 1 tablespoon and then season to your preference. Seafood tends to toughen (especially shrimp) if it cooks too long, so it's best to add the seafood after the simmering process is finished and the soup has cooled. I have also successfully used lobster and crabmeat as seafood choices.

8 servings

*2 tablespoons neutral oil (expeller-pressed canola, high-oleic safflower, or
  sunflower oil)*
½ cup onion, chopped
½ cup red pepper, chopped
2 cloves garlic, minced
2 tablespoons chili seasoning
1 can (28 ounces) fire-roasted diced tomatoes
2 cans (15 ounces each) cannellini beans
¼ cup mild salsa
3 tablespoons Worcestershire sauce
¾ teaspoon salt
1 pound cooked crawfish meat, thawed
1 pound large shrimp, cooked and cut into bite-sized pieces
Sour cream if desired

1. In a large pot over moderate heat, heat the oil and sauté the onion, red pepper, and garlic until tender. Add the chili seasoning and cook for about 1 minute. Add the tomatoes, cannellini beans, salsa, Worcestershire sauce, and salt. Simmer for about 1 hour. When the chili has cooled, add the crawfish meat and shrimp. Cover and refrigerate overnight.
2. Allow the chili to come to room temperature before heating. Serve hot. Pass the sour cream to your guests if desired.

CREAMY LOBSTER SOUP

Despite it being the first day of spring, it was chilly the day we hosted Nick's lifelong friend to celebrate his birthday. I didn't know that when he awakened that morning, he announced to his wife he wanted to eat lobster for his birthday. I was thrilled that I'd delivered his wish, however unbeknownst. I served bowls of hot soup, a baby arugula salad that was topped with roasted asparagus and cast-iron honey-glazed cornbread (page 115); for dessert I poked birthday candles into rhubarb pie (page 220). A springtime birthday meal extraordinaire.

8 servings

4 lobster tails (about 8 to 10 ounces each), about 2 cups
4 tablespoons butter
2 cups onion, finely chopped
2 cups celery, finely chopped
1 package (8 ounces) or about 8 to 10 medium-sized white mushrooms, sliced
4 tablespoons unbleached all-purpose flour
2 cups chicken broth
2 cups milk
2 cups heavy cream
2 cups water
4 vegetable bouillon cubes
4 tablespoons cooking sherry
A few grindings of black pepper
¼ cup fresh parsley, minced

1. In a large pot, steam the lobster tails until cooked through, about 8 to 10 minutes. Transfer the lobster tails to a cutting board and allow to cool. When they are cool enough to handle, remove the shells and cut the lobster into bite-sized pieces.

2. In a large pot over moderate heat, melt the butter and sauté the onion, celery, and mushrooms until tender. Add the flour, 1 tablespoon at a time (the onion/celery mixture will grab the flour quickly). Slowly add the chicken broth, stirring constantly. Reduce the heat and add the milk, heavy cream, water, bouillon cubes, cooking sherry, pepper, and parsley. Add the lobster. Cover and simmer until heated through. Serve immediately.

SHRIMP AND COCONUT SOUP WITH ROASTED CORN AND SWEET POTATO

Maybe you scraped fresh corn off corn cobs when it was in season and have an abundant supply stocked in the freezer to use throughout the winter months. If not, frozen corn kernels will work with nearly the same flavor results. I like to serve this hearty, healthy, flavor-charged soup on a cold wintry night with slices of good crusty bread. Coconut milk naturally separates and hardens—it will become fluid when heated. Shake the can well before opening and stir until fully blended before adding to the remaining ingredients.

6 to 8 servings

2 cups fresh or frozen corn kernels, thawed if frozen
Olive oil
Coarse salt
1 tablespoon coconut oil
1 teaspoon cumin
1 teaspoon curry powder
1 teaspoon turmeric powder
1 cup sweet onion, chopped
3 cloves garlic, chopped
1 large sweet potato, peeled and diced
2 cups water
1 vegetable bouillon cube
1 can (14 ounces) fire-roasted diced tomatoes
1 can (4 ounces) chopped green chiles
1 can (14 ounces) coconut milk
2 cups cooked shrimp, cut into bite-sized pieces
Fresh snipped chives (garnish)

1. Set the oven temperature to broil.
2. In a medium bowl, toss the corn with the olive oil and salt. Transfer the corn to a parchment-lined rimmed baking sheet and broil until the corn is chestnut brown in spots.

3. In a large pot, heat the oil over moderate heat. Add the cumin, curry powder, and turmeric, and cook for about 1 minute or until fragrant. Add the onion and sauté until translucent. Add the garlic, sweet potato, water, and bouillon cube. Cover the pot and bring the mixture to a gentle boil and cook until the sweet potato is tender.

4. Add the tomatoes, green chiles, coconut milk, and shrimp. Simmer until heated through. Serve immediately.

CUCUMBER AND CRAB SOUP

The base of this soup is velvety smooth, making the bite-sized morsels of cucumber and crab a delightful contrast of textures. Serve with good-quality bread and a tossed salad.

6 servings

6 tablespoons butter
2 cups onion, chopped
6 tablespoons unbleached all-purpose flour
5 cups water
3 vegetable bouillon cubes
2 medium (about 3 cups) cucumbers, peeled, seeded, and cubed
1 cup milk
1 pound (16 ounces) lump crabmeat
Fresh snipped chives (garnish)

1. Melt the butter in a large pot over medium heat. Add the onion and sauté until tender. Gradually add the flour, 1 tablespoon at a time, whisking after each addition. While continuing to whisk, gradually add the water, 1 cup at a time.
2. Add the bouillon cubes, and stir until the cubes have dissolved into the mixture. Add the cucumbers, cover, and bring the mixture to a boil. Reduce the heat and simmer for 10 to 15 minutes, or until the cucumbers are tender. Add the milk and crabmeat. Cook over low heat until heated through. Serve immediately.

CURRIED PUMPKIN SOUP WITH MUSHROOMS

Here is a twist from the norm where I've combined curry, pumpkin, and mushrooms. This unlikely combination creates a delightful mild and earthy flavor. It's a wonderful soup to serve when summer gives way to autumn.

6 servings

4 tablespoons butter
1 large onion, chopped
1 package (10 ounces) or about 13 to 15 medium-sized white mushrooms, sliced
2½ teaspoons curry powder
3 teaspoons all-purpose flour
3 cups water
2 vegetable bouillon cubes
1 can (16 ounces) pure pumpkin
1 tablespoon honey
1 teaspoon salt
A few grindings of black pepper
1 cup cream
Fresh minced parsley (garnish)

1. Melt the butter in a large pot over medium heat. Add the onion and mushrooms, and sauté until the onions are translucent and the mushrooms are tender.
2. Add the curry powder and cook for about 1 minute. Sprinkle the flour over the mixture and stir to combine. Add the water and bouillon cubes and stir until they dissolve. Add the pumpkin, honey, salt, and pepper, and cook until the mixture is heated through. Stir in the cream and simmer until the soup is hot. Serve immediately.

GINGERED BUTTERNUT SQUASH SOUP WITH COCONUT

For those of you who have come to know me, you've learned how I love to combine ginger, coconut, and vegetables. This flavor combination delivers on many levels and has an oh-wow, jaw-dropping kind of effect on people. Serve for lunch or dinner, or as a first course for a sit-down dinner party.

8 servings

4 tablespoons butter
1 cup onion, chopped
1 cup celery, chopped
1 apple, unpeeled and chopped
2 teaspoons powdered ginger
5 cups water
3 vegetable bouillon cubes
1 cinnamon stick
4½ pounds butternut squash, peeled and cut into bite-sized pieces
1½ teaspoons salt
A few grindings of black pepper
1 can (14 ounces) coconut milk

1. Heat the butter in a large pot over medium-high heat. Add the onion, celery, and apple, and cook until tender. Add the ginger and cook for about 1 minute. Add the water, bouillon cubes, cinnamon stick, butternut squash, salt, and pepper. Cover and bring the mixture to a boil. Reduce the heat and simmer until the butternut squash is tender.

2. Remove from heat and discard the cinnamon stick. Allow the mixture to cool slightly before transferring to a food processor or blender. Purée the butternut squash mixture in batches until silky smooth. Add the coconut milk to the last batch to be puréed. Transfer all puréed soup back into the original large pot and stir until well combined. Serve hot.

CREAMY WILD MUSHROOM SOUP WITH TURMERIC

If you're a fan of mushrooms, you will love this soup. I use a combination of beech, royal trumpet, and shitake mushrooms.

4 servings

2 tablespoons butter
1 cup leeks, sliced
⅓ cup shallots, sliced (1 large)
1 package (5 ounces) assorted wild mushrooms, chopped
1 cup carrots, julienned
2 tablespoons unbleached all-purpose flour
2 cups milk
1 vegetable bouillon cube
1 teaspoon turmeric powder
Several grindings of black pepper
2 tablespoons cooking sherry
1 cup frozen peas, thawed

1. In a medium pot over moderate heat, melt the butter and sauté the leeks and shallots until tender. Add the mushrooms and the carrots and sauté, stirring frequently until the mushrooms are tender. Add the flour 1 tablespoon at a time and, working quickly, whisk the flour with the ingredients. Lower the heat and add the milk in a steady stream, stirring until the flour has melded with the milk.

2. Cover and simmer for 5 to 10 minutes or until the carrots are tender. Add the bouillon cube, turmeric, black pepper, sherry, and thawed peas. Cook until heated though. Serve immediately.

VEGETABLE CHOWDER WITH CHEESE TORTELLINI

I first served this at a dinner party we were hosting. Tasters proclaimed it to be the tastiest chowder they had ever eaten. It needs nothing more than a tossed green salad, hot rolls slathered with butter, good company, and a nice bottle of wine. Just about any vegetable works in this recipe. I've experimented using any combination of broccoli, cauliflower, spinach, peas, green beans, and corn kernels with great results. Use the harvest as your guide and design whatever combination of vegetables are in season. If you don't eat this in one sitting, the tortellini will swell over time, so you may need to add more liquid.

6 servings

1 package (10 ounces) cheese tortellini
2 tablespoons butter
1 package (8 ounces) or about 6 to 8 medium-sized white mushrooms, chopped
1 cup leeks, sliced
1 cup celery, sliced
1 cup red pepper, chopped
1 cup carrots, julienned
4 cups water
2 vegetable bouillon cubes
¼ cup fresh parsley, minced
1 teaspoon salt
A few grindings of black pepper
1 cup heavy cream

1. Bring a large pot of water to a boil. When the water boils, cook the tortellini according to the package directions. Drain and set aside.
2. Melt the butter in a large pot over moderate heat and sauté the mushrooms, leeks, celery, red pepper, and carrots. Cook for about 5 minutes, stirring frequently. Add the water and bring the mixture to a boil. Cover and cook for about 5 minutes or until the vegetables are tender.
3. Add the parsley and bouillon cubes and stir until the cubes dissolve. Add the salt and pepper and cooked tortellini. Stir in the cream. Simmer the chowder until heated through. Serve immediately.

CREAM OF TURNIP SOUP WITH PUMPERNICKEL CROUTONS

The plan for the turnips I picked up at the farmers' market was to make one of our favorite turnip recipes, honey-buttered peppered turnips and sweet peas (page 99), to serve with our baked chicken. Instead, I turned the beautiful rustic-looking white balls with their lavender-colored tops into this mellow-tasting comfort-food soup. Its pearly color contrasts beautifully with the punctuation of pumpernickel croutons. Later, I served it as a first course on Thanksgiving, and everyone loved it—even the kids!

8 servings

2 tablespoons butter
1 medium onion, chopped
4 to 5 medium turnips, peeled and cubed
1 medium russet or Yukon Gold potato, peeled and cubed
3 cup water
3 vegetable bouillon cubes
¼ cup cooking sherry
¼ cup heavy cream
2½ cups pumpernickel bread, cubed
Fresh snipped chives (garnish)

1. In a large pot over moderate heat, melt the butter. Add the onion and sauté until the onions are translucent. Add the turnips, potatoes, and water, and bring the mixture to a boil. Cover and reduce the heat to simmer and cook for 20 to 30 minutes, until the turnips and potatoes are tender. Remove from heat and allow the mixture to cool slightly.
2. Preheat the oven to 350°F.
3. While the potatoes and turnips are cooking, prepare the pumpernickel croutons. In a large bowl, toss the pumpernickel cubes with the olive oil. Transfer the cubes to a parchment-lined rimmed baking sheet and bake for 10 to 15 minutes or until crispy.
4. In a food processor or blender, purée the soup in batches. Transfer the puréed batches into a large bowl. In the last batch to be puréed, add the sherry and cream. Transfer all the puréed soup back into the original large pot and stir to blend. Simmer the soup until heated through. Garnish bowls of soup with pumpernickel croutons and chives. Serve immediately.

COCONUT BLACK BEAN SOUP WITH MANGO AND AVOCADO SALSA

For the salsa to impart the most flavor, the mango and avocado should be perfectly ripe. Taste-testers' favorite pairing with this hearty soup is the hot-from-the-oven cast-iron honey-glazed cornbread (page 115). Coconut milk naturally separates and hardens—it will become fluid when heated. Shake the can well before opening and stir until fully blended before adding to the red curry paste mixture.

6 servings

1 tablespoon coconut oil
1 cup onion, chopped
3 cloves garlic, minced
2 teaspoons cumin
3 teaspoons red curry paste
1 can (14 ounces) coconut milk
½ cup chunky natural peanut butter
2 cans (15 ounces each) black beans
1½ cups carrots, julienned
1 teaspoon salt
Several grindings of black pepper
1 avocado, cut into bite-sized pieces
1 mango, cut into bite-sized pieces
1 tablespoon olive oil
1 teaspoon rice vinegar

1. In a large skillet, heat the oil over moderate heat and sauté the onion until tender. Add the garlic and sauté for 1 to 2 minutes. Add the cumin and sauté, stirring constantly for about 1 minute. Add the red curry paste and stir until the paste is blended with the other ingredients. Add the coconut milk and peanut butter. Reduce the heat and stir until the ingredients are well blended. Add the black beans, carrots, salt, and pepper. Cover and simmer for 10 to 15 minutes, until the carrots are tender. Simmer over a low heat until serving time.

2. Prepare the mango and avocado salsa just before serving. In a medium bowl, combine the avocado with the mango. Add the olive oil and vinegar, and gently stir to combine.

3. Ladle the hot soup into bowls and pass the mango and avocado salsa to your guests.

MUSHROOM SOUP WITH SPINACH TORTELLINI

A simple and great wintry soup to offer when not much is in season locally and we can rely on mushrooms (available year-round) and traditionally preserved tomatoes. Serve with crusty bread accompanied with olive oil for dipping.

4 to 6 servings

1 package (10 ounces) fresh spinach tortellini
2 tablespoons neutral oil (expeller-pressed canola, high-oleic safflower, or sunflower oil)
1 cup onions, chopped
1 package (8 ounces) or about 8 to 10 medium-sized white mushrooms, sliced
3 cups water
2 vegetable bouillon cubes
1 can (14 ounces) fire-roasted diced tomatoes
⅛ cup cooking sherry
½ teaspoon salt
A few grindings of black pepper
2 tablespoons fresh parsley, minced

1. Bring a large pot of water to a boil. When the water boils, cook the tortellini according to the package directions. Drain and set aside.
2. While you're waiting for the water to boil to cook the tortellini, start cooking the vegetables. Heat the oil in a large pot over moderate heat, and sauté the onions and mushrooms for about 5 minutes or until tender. Add the water and bouillon cubes and stir until they dissolve. Add the tomatoes, sherry, salt, pepper, tortellini, and parsley. Simmer until heated through. Serve immediately.

GINGERED TURNIP SOUP WITH COCONUT

Another fine combination of ginger and coconut with the addition of the humble turnip. It's a fun soup to serve because no one can guess turnips are the primary ingredient, and then tasters can't believe how delicious it is.

6 servings

1 cup milk
1 cup water
1 vegetable bouillon cube
4 cups turnip, peeled and cut into chunks
1 cup white onion, cut into chunks
1 teaspoon salt
1 teaspoon ground ginger
½ cup raw slivered almonds
1 can (14 ounces) coconut milk
Ground turmeric (garnish)

1. In a large pot, combine the milk, water, and vegetable cube. Bring the mixture to a gentle boil over moderate heat. Add the turnips, onion, salt, ginger, and almonds. Bring the mixture to a gentle boil. Cover and reduce the heat to simmer (mixture should be rumbling), and cook for 30 to 40 minutes or until the turnips are tender. (When milk is brought to a boil and simmered as it is in this recipe, the milk curdles or "breaks." When you uncover the pot, the mixture doesn't look very appetizing, but once you blend it, it turns as smooth as cream.)
2. Remove from heat and allow the mixture to cool slightly before transferring to a food processor or blender. Purée the turnip mixture in batches until silky smooth.
3. Add the coconut milk to the last batch to be puréed. Transfer all the puréed soup back into the original large pot and stir until well combined. Cook until heated through. Garnish bowls of soup with ground turmeric. Serve immediately.

GREEN BEAN CASSEROLE SOUP

This soup is as delicious as the famous and wildly popular 1950s classic green bean casserole that was served at just about everybody's holiday table—and still is. I generally don't experiment with such reliable pleasures, but I couldn't resist turning this classic can't-get-enough casserole's ingredients into a delicious pot of soup using fresh ingredients instead of tinned. More exotic mushrooms, specifically a combination of beech, royal trumpet, and shitake, replace the white button mushrooms. Thinly sliced shallots that are sautéed until crispy replace the traditional french-fried onions—the topping for the green bean casserole. Tradition evolved! The result is a mouth-watering, delicious soup you will be proud to serve.

4 servings

3 tablespoons butter
1 package (8 ounces) assorted mushrooms, sliced
3 tablespoons flour
2 cups water
1 vegetable bouillon cube
1 cup heavy cream
2 cups green beans, cooked and cut into bite-sized pieces
4 tablespoons cooking sherry
½ teaspoon salt, or to taste
A few grindings of black pepper
4 shallots, thinly sliced
Buttermilk
Unbleached all-purpose flour
Neutral oil (expeller-pressed canola, high-oleic safflower, or sunflower oil)

1. In a medium pot over moderate heat, melt the butter and sauté the mushrooms until tender. Add the flour 1 tablespoon at a time, whisking well after each addition. Add the water 1 cup at a time, stirring well to incorporate the ingredients. Add the bouillon cube and stir until it dissolves. Add the cream, green beans, sherry, salt, and pepper, and stir to combine. Simmer the soup while you prepare the shallots.
2. In a medium bowl, place enough buttermilk to coat the shallots. Dredge the shallots in the buttermilk. Transfer the shallots to another bowl and dust them generously and evenly with flour.

45

3. Cover the bottom of a sauté pan with oil. Heat the oil over moderately high heat and sauté the shallots until chestnut brown.

4. Ladle the soup into serving bowls and top each bowl with the crispy shallots. Serve immediately.

GINGERED COCONUT AND CELERY SOUP

A delicious creamy soup that won't disappoint! I love to serve it as a first course, because it sets the mood for a great beginning to a wonderful dinner with family or friends.

6 servings

1 cup milk
1 cup water
1 vegetable bouillon cube
4 cups celery, cut into chunks
1 cup white onion, cut into chunks
1 teaspoon salt
1 teaspoon ground ginger
½ cup raw slivered almonds
1 can (14 ounces) coconut milk

1. Combine the milk, water, and bouillon cube in a large pot. Bring the mixture to a boil over moderate heat. Add the celery, onion, salt, ginger, and almonds. Cover and reduce the heat to simmer (mixture should be rumbling), and cook for 30 to 40 minutes or until the celery is tender. (When milk is brought to a boil and simmered as it is in this recipe, the milk curdles or "breaks." When you uncover the pot, the mixture doesn't look very appetizing, but once you blend it, it turns as smooth as cream.)
2. Remove from heat and allow the mixture to cool slightly before transferring to a food processor or blender. Purée the celery mixture in batches until silky smooth.
3. Add the coconut milk to the last batch to be puréed. Transfer all the puréed soup back into original large pot and stir until well combined. Cook until heated through. Serve immediately.

WINTER SOLSTICE SOUP

The winter solstice falls four days before Christmas. It is the shortest day of the year and the day we receive the least amount of sunlight. For me, it's the beginning of the time of year when meals are made up mostly of soups, casseroles, and one-pot meals, each served with piping hot home-baked breads—the kind of warming, hearty foods we usually partake of in front of a roaring fire. With Christmas just four days away and all the holiday flurry, I'm ready for the onslaught of the holiday festivities and can't think of a more inviting and healthy soup—amidst all the overindulgence—to enjoy and celebrate on the evening of the winter solstice. This soup ages beautifully; it's better made the day before you plan to serve it.

6 servings

3 cups water
1 cup red lentils
1 can (14.5 ounces) fire-roasted tomatoes
1 can (14 ounces) coconut milk
2 tablespoons red curry paste
2 tablespoons tahini
2 teaspoons salt
2 teaspoons coriander
1 teaspoon turmeric
½ teaspoon ground cumin
½ teaspoon paprika

1. In a large pot over high heat, bring the water to a boil. Add the lentils, partially cover the pot, and reduce the heat to a simmer. Cook until the lentils are tender, about 20 minutes.
2. Add the tomatoes, coconut milk, red curry paste, tahini, salt, coriander, turmeric, ground cumin, and paprika, and stir until ingredients are fully incorporated. Simmer the soup for about a half hour to allow the flavors to mingle.
3. Allow the soup to cool before covering and refrigerating overnight.
4. Bring the soup to room temperature before simmering until hot. Serve immediately.

What's for Dinner?

BEEF, LAMB, PORK
CHICKEN AND TURKEY
SEAFOOD
VEGETARIAN

Evening, the time of day when we all come together and the day draws to a close, is a time to wind down and partake of a meal with family and friends. For every season—the chill of a blustery winter, the promise of budding spring, the swelter of summer, and the glory of fall colors—this chapter has recipes that range from easy and comforting to elegant and impressive.

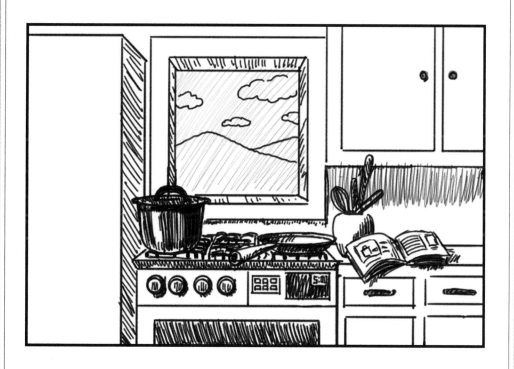

RECIPE INDEX

BEEF, LAMB, PORK

Cast-Iron New York Strip Steak 52

Moist and Tender Roast Beef 53

Beef, Cheese, and Black Bean Enchiladas 54

American-Style Meatloaf with Pineapple Glaze 55

Creamed Chipped Beef with Mushrooms 56

Leg of Lamb Roast Stuffed with Spinach, Feta, and Pine Nuts 57-58

Pork Tenderloin with Roasted Coffee and Allspice 59

Egg Noodles with Creamed Spinach and Bacon 60

CHICKEN AND TURKEY

Savory-Sweet Apricot Chicken 61-62

Maple Dijon Glazed Chicken 63

Curried Cinnamon Orange Marmalade Tomatoes with Chicken and Hearts of Palm 64

Chicken, Vegetables, and Brown Rice Pasta with Red Curry Coconut Sauce 65-66

Moist and Delicious Holiday Turkey 67-68

SEAFOOD

Old Bay Crab Cakes 69

Herbed Trout with Fried Carrots 70

Creamy Shrimp and Pasta with Arugula Pesto 71

Lemon-Marinated Catfish with Artichoke Hearts and Kalamata Olives 72

Apricot Tomatoes with Hearts of Palm, Shrimp, and Feta 73

Baked Cod with Toasted Coconut and Pineapple Salsa 74

VEGETARIAN

Quinoa Cheeseburgers with Curried Cucumber Yogurt Sauce 75-76

Cheesy Eggplant, Bean, and Vegetable Casserole 77

Creamy Lemon Penne Pasta with Broccoli 78

Herbed Cabbage and Mushroom Pie 79-80

Palak Paneer 81

Wild Porcini Mushroom Lasagna 82

CAST-IRON NEW YORK STRIP STEAK

It took a few times before I perfected cooking a New York strip steak on the stovetop in my beloved cast-iron skillet. Once I achieved it, the steaks turned out similar to the steaks in the really good steak houses. Before I cook the steaks, I season the meat with one of my favorite seasoning blends from A.A. Borsari, a delicious blend of sea salt, garlic, basil, rosemary, black pepper, and nutmeg that works well with beef. See the Product Reference Guide (page 233) or use your favorite seasoning.

1 steak per person

1½-inch-thick New York strip steaks, at room temperature
High-heat oil (peanut, sesame, or sunflower oil)
Steak seasoning
Butter

1. Preheat the oven to 400°F.
2. Coat a cast-iron skillet with oil. When the oven has preheated, place the skillet in the oven for 15 minutes.
3. Coat the steaks evenly with oil. Just prior to placing the steaks in the hot skillet, season them generously with steak seasoning. After the skillet has been in the oven for 15 minutes, remove and place the skillet on the stovetop.
4. Set the stovetop temperature dial to medium high (if your stove dials are numbered, set the dial to just between 6 and 8), and cook the steaks for 5 minutes. Turn the steaks and set the stovetop dial to medium (or just between 4 and 6), and cook for an additional 5 minutes. (These cooking times and temperatures are for 1½-inch-thick steaks cooked medium rare. Adjust the cooking times based on your preference.)
5. Remove the steaks and transfer them to a serving platter. Top each steak with a tablespoon or more of butter. Let them rest for about 5 minutes before serving.

MOIST AND TENDER ROAST BEEF

Thoughts of roast beef take me down Memory Lane, making the nostalgia element just as significant as the dish itself. Roast beef was often our family's Sunday night dinner, served with creamy mashed potatoes, succotash, and one of my mother's family-famous salads with the best homemade croutons. Roast beef was popular then, and, above all, it was one of my dad's favorite cuts of beef. Like most cuts of beef, perfection lies in it being perfectly cooked. And he was a stickler for a medium-rare roast. After many attempts, my mother finally nailed the cooking time. Her method is a great way to cook the most flavorful and tender roast beef. Follow the directions exactly and you will have a perfectly cooked (medium-rare) roast. Be sure to remove the roast from the refrigerator about 2 hours prior to cooking. I season the beef with A.A. Borsari Seasoned Salt (see Product Reference Guide, page 233). It's a delicious blend known as the caviar of seasoned salts. Or use your favorite seasoning for beef.

12 servings

1 (3-pound) beef eye-of-round roast
Olive oil
A.A. Borsari Seasoned Salt

1. Preheat the oven to 500°F. Once the oven has reached temperature, leave it on for 20 minutes.
2. Rub the roast with olive oil and generously cover with salt seasoning.
3. Place the roast fat side up on a rack in a shallow baking pan. Place it in the oven and immediately reduce the temperature to 475°F. Cook for 21 minutes. (Regardless of the size of the roast, cooking for 7 minutes per pound is the perfect formula.)
4. Turn off the oven and leave the roast in for 18 minutes per pound. (Do not open the door to peek.) When the cooking time is complete, remove the roast from the baking pan, transfer it to a platter, and let it stand for 20 minutes. Thinly slice and serve immediately.

Beef, Cheese, and Black Bean Enchiladas

When you have a hankering for Mexican-style fare, this American-influenced dish will satisfy your craving.

6 servings

1 tablespoon neutral oil (expeller-pressed canola, high-oleic safflower, or sunflower oil)
1 cup onion, chopped
1 pound ground beef
4 teaspoons chili powder
2 teaspoons cumin powder
1 teaspoon oregano
1 teaspoon salt
¼ teaspoon red pepper flakes
1 can (15 ounces) black beans, drained
2½ cups shredded Monterey Jack cheese
6 (7-inch) soft flour tortillas
1 can (14 ounces) enchilada sauce
Sides of sour cream and guacamole

1. Preheat the oven to 350°F.
2. Coat the bottom and sides of a 13 x 9 x 2-inch baking dish with cooking spray.
3. In a large skillet over medium heat, heat the oil and sauté the onion until tender. Add the ground beef and cook until the beef has browned. Add the chili powder, cumin, oregano, salt, red pepper, and beans. Stir until well combined.
4. Working with one tortilla at a time, top the center of each tortilla shell with about ¼ cup of cheese and evenly distribute the beef/bean mixture over the top of the cheese. Roll the tortilla shell and place seam side down into the prepared baking dish.
5. Top the tortilla shells with any of the leftover beef/bean mixture. Pour the enchilada sauce evenly over the tortilla shells and top the sauce with the remaining cheese.
6. Bake uncovered for 45 minutes or until bubbly. Serve immediately and pass the sour cream and guacamole to your guests.

AMERICAN-STYLE MEATLOAF WITH PINEAPPLE GLAZE

I love the aroma that wafts through the house when meatloaf is doing its magic in the oven. A savory perfume so strong and inviting, it continues to strike a decades-long comfort-food chord—a flavor flashback. (As a child, the smell worked wonders on distracting me from concentrating on schoolwork.) This meatloaf satisfies on many levels. For starters, it's cozy-up comfort food, and the flavor from the sweet pineapple preserves and the zesty horseradish glaze marries beautifully with the meatloaf's ingredients. It begs to be served with traditional accompaniments like creamy mashed potatoes and buttered peas and carrots. Recommendations for brands of pineapple preserves and horseradish can be found in the Product Reference Guide (page 233).

8 servings

2 pounds ground beef
1 cup carrots, shredded
1 cup onion, chopped
2 eggs
½ cup quick-cooking oatmeal
1 teaspoon salt
Several grindings of black pepper
½ cup pineapple preserves
½ cup ketchup
2 tablespoons prepared horseradish
1 tablespoon Worcestershire sauce
1 teaspoon Dijon-style mustard

1. Preheat the oven to 375°F.
2. In a large bowl, combine the ground beef with the carrots and the onion.
3. In a medium bowl, combine the eggs with the oatmeal, salt, and pepper. Whisk until well blended. Add the oatmeal mixture to the meat mixture and mix until the ingredients are evenly distributed.
4. Transfer the mixture to a 13 x 9 x 2-inch baking dish and shape it into a rectangular or oval loaf.
5. In a small saucepan, combine the pineapple preserves, ketchup, horseradish, Worcestershire sauce, and mustard. Mix until well blended. Spoon the pineapple glaze mixture over the meatloaf and bake uncovered for 45 minutes. Serve immediately.

CREAMED CHIPPED BEEF WITH MUSHROOMS

When we were kids, my mother prepared various dishes using chipped beef (aka dried beef), and we relished every one. We especially loved the creamed chipped beef that she would make for breakfast that covered slices of homemade toast. Sometimes she would make a savory version, adding mushrooms and seasoning the mixture with sherry and ground black pepper. She would serve it for dinner on cold wintry nights over homemade bread, and we savored every morsel. I also serve it spooned over homemade toast, but it's hard to resist spooning this mushroom-infused, salty, creamy mixture on the nooks and crannies of an English muffin.

4 servings

4 tablespoons butter
1 package (8 ounces) or about 8 to 10 medium-sized white mushrooms, sliced
1 package (4 ounces) chipped beef, chopped
4 tablespoons unbleached all-purpose flour
2½ cups milk
1 tablespoon cooking sherry
A few grindings of black pepper
8 slices of good-quality bread or 4 English muffins, split in half

1. In a medium pan, over moderate heat melt the butter and sauté the mushrooms until they are soft. Add the chipped beef and sauté for 1 to 2 minutes. Add the flour 1 tablespoon at a time, stirring well after each addition. Slowly add the milk, stirring constantly, and reduce the heat when the mixture begins to thicken. Add the cooking sherry and black pepper.
2. Toast the bread or English muffins to your liking. Spoon creamed chipped beef over toast or muffins. Serve immediately.

Leg of Lamb Roast Stuffed with Spinach, Feta, and Pine Nuts

I had been wavering about what to serve for a dinner we were hosting for friends we see once a year. Our annual gathering is special, and I think lamb falls into the special dinner category. Part of what makes this roast so flavorful is a special blend of seasonings from A.A. Borsari, a unique blend of gourmet salts known as the caviar of seasoned salts (see Product Reference Guide, page 233). Plan accordingly; the roast needs to come to room temperature, and the sun-dried tomatoes need to soak for an hour.

6 to 8 servings

2½ pounds boneless leg of lamb roast
¼ cup sun-dried tomatoes
½ cup boiling water
6 cloves of garlic, unpeeled
3 tablespoons neutral oil (expeller-pressed canola, high-oleic safflower, or
*   sunflower oil)*
1 cup onion, thinly sliced
16 ounces frozen chopped spinach, defrosted, drained, and squeezed dry
⅛ cup pine nuts
¼ cup feta cheese, crumbled
Olive oil
A.A. Borsari Seasoned Salt
½ cup red wine

1. Remove the lamb from the refrigerator about 2 hours prior to cooking.
2. Place the sun-dried tomatoes in a small bowl. Pour the boiling water over them and let them soak for 1 hour. Drain the tomatoes (you can reserve the broth and add to a soup stock or to pasta water), and finely chop.
3. Preheat the oven to 300°F.
4. Roast the garlic cloves for 5 to 10 minutes or until soft. When the cloves are cool enough to handle, remove the skin and roughly chop.

5. Heat 1 tablespoon of neutral oil over moderate heat and sauté the onion until soft and slightly brown in spots. Add the sun-dried tomatoes, garlic, and spinach to the onion. Stir until fully combined

6. Preheat the oven to 425°F.

7. Coat the entire roast with olive oil. Season the non-fatty side with seasoned salt and press the seasoning mixture into the roast. Transfer the spinach mixture to the roast and spread the mixture evenly over it. Scatter the pine nuts and feta over the spinach and press them into it.

8. Roll the roast and tie it together in several places using kitchen twine.

9. Heat 1 to 2 tablespoons of neutral oil in a large skillet over moderately high heat and sear the roast on all sides. Transfer the lamb, fat side up, to a parchment-lined rimmed baking dish that's been fitted with a wire rack.

10. Add the wine to the hot skillet and scrape the bottom to get any of the mixture that fell out of the roast. Pour the wine mixture over the roast.

11. Cook the lamb at 425°F for 20 minutes. Reduce the oven temperature to 325°F and cook for another 30 minutes for medium rare or 40 minutes for medium. Let the lamb stand for 20 to 30 minutes before slicing.

PORK TENDERLOIN WITH ROASTED COFFEE AND ALLSPICE

Flavor boosters like allspice, chili powder, and cinnamon impart a wonderful flavor to pork. This simple recipe pairs well with unembellished sides like roasted potatoes and a steamed seasonal vegetable medley like carrots, cauliflower, and peas for an easy weeknight meal.

About 6 to 8 servings

2 tablespoons freshly ground coffee beans
2 teaspoons brown sugar
1 teaspoon salt
1 teaspoon allspice
1 teaspoon chili powder
¼ teaspoon ground cinnamon
2 tablespoons olive oil
2 (about 1¼ pounds each) pork tenderloins

1. Preheat the oven to 375°F.
2. In a small bowl, combine the ground coffee with the brown sugar, salt, allspice, chili powder, and cinnamon.
3. Rub both tenderloins with the olive oil and cover them with the roasted coffee rub.
4. Place a rack over a rimmed baking pan, and place the tenderloins on the rack. Cook for 45 minutes. Allow the tenderloins to cool before carving into desired-size slices.

EGG NOODLES WITH CREAMED SPINACH AND BACON

I called from the kitchen and asked, "How is it?" In unison, the taste-testers said, "The first bite will let you know. Comfort food extraordinaire!"

4 servings

3 cups raw egg noodles
1 tablespoon neutral oil (expeller-pressed canola, high-oleic safflower, or sunflower oil)
1 slice Canadian bacon, finely chopped
3 garlic cloves, crushed
½ cup mascarpone cheese
½ cup heavy cream
A pinch of ground nutmeg
10 ounces frozen chopped spinach, defrosted, drained, and squeezed dry
Salt and pepper, to taste

1. Fill a large pot three-quarters full with water. Add salt if desired. Bring the water to a boil over high heat. Add the egg noodles and cook according to the package directions.
2. While the noodles are cooking, prepare the cream sauce. In a large skillet, heat the oil over medium-high heat. Cook the Canadian bacon for a few minutes or until lightly browned. Reduce the heat to medium-low, add the crushed garlic, and cook for about 1 minute or until fragrant. Add the mascarpone, cream, and nutmeg. Whisk until smooth and well combined. Add the spinach, and stir to combine. Season the mixture with salt and pepper.
3. When the noodles have finished cooking, drain, and immediately add them to the cream sauce. Stir until well combined and heated through. Serve immediately.

SAVORY-SWEET APRICOT CHICKEN

The inspiration for this combination came from the wildly popular recipe for curried cinnamon orange marmalade tomatoes with chicken and hearts of palm (page 64), where savory and sweet come together in absolute harmony. The first time I served this dish, I marveled as dinner party guests devoured it, observing that it was the first item on the plate to disappear. Plan accordingly; marinating overnight is essential. It allows all the savory-sweet ingredients to mingle. Cooking them with the skin on and bone in helps give the chicken its rich flavor. I look for small chicken breasts. If I can get only the larger versions, I cook the dish, allow it to cool, remove the bone, and slice the breasts into desired-size slices, return the slices to the dish, and reheat the chicken. This vibrant-tasting dish is delicious served with steamed rice and an unembellished steamed vegetable like green beans.

6 to 8 servings

1 head of garlic, peeled
½ cup olive oil
3 tablespoons dried oregano
½ cup red wine vinegar
1 tablespoon coarse salt
1 teaspoon pepper
1 cup dried apricots, chopped
½ cup Spanish green olives, chopped
¼ cup capers plus 1 tablespoon caper juice
4 bay leaves
1 cup white wine or cooking wine
1 cup brown sugar
About 3½ pounds chicken breasts, bone in, skin on

1. Place the garlic cloves in a food processor and add ¼ cup of olive oil. Process until nearly smooth. Transfer the garlic/olive oil mixture to a 15 x 10 x 2-inch baking dish. Add the remaining olive oil, oregano, vinegar, salt, and pepper. Whisk the mixture until well combined. Add the apricots, olives, capers, caper juice, bay leaves, wine, and brown sugar. Stir to combine.
2. Place the chicken breasts, skin side down, over the marinade. Cover and refrigerate overnight.

3. Allow the chicken to come to room temperature—1 to 2 hours prior to cooking.

4. Preheat the oven to 350°F.

5. Turn the chicken breasts over, skin side up, and bake uncovered for 1 to 1½ hours or until the chicken is cooked through—basting halfway through cooking time. Just before serving, spoon the essence over the chicken. Transfer any reserved marinade to a bowl and serve with the chicken. Serve immediately.

MAPLE DIJON GLAZED CHICKEN

Nick dubbed this delicious combination "Elemental Pleasures." It's a no-fuss recipe and one you will come back to time and time again—go-to weeknight fare. Use any desired assortment of chicken pieces. The flavor of this dish is so pronounced, I like to accompany the chicken with steamed rice and unembellished vegetables.

4 servings

½ cup Dijon-style mustard
¼ cup pure maple syrup
1 tablespoon rice vinegar
3½ pounds chicken, bone in, skin on
Salt and freshly ground black pepper

1. Preheat the oven to 450°F.
2. Cover the bottom and sides of a rimmed baking sheet with parchment paper.
3. In a large bowl, combine the mustard, maple syrup, and vinegar. Add the chicken pieces and toss them with the mustard sauce.
4. Transfer the chicken to the prepared baking sheet and season with salt and pepper. Bake for 40 minutes. Baste the chicken with any extra sauce halfway through the cooking time. Transfer the chicken to a serving platter. Serve immediately.

CURRIED CINNAMON ORANGE MARMALADE TOMATOES WITH CHICKEN AND HEARTS OF PALM

One of my catering clients requested chicken with a sweet tomato sauce to serve to her family for Christmas Eve dinner. I didn't have such a recipe and set out to deliver her wish. I started by using the popular recipe for orange marmalade tomatoes from *This Book Cooks*. I added cooked chicken pieces to the tomatoes and slices of hearts of palm. It is an amazing combination of flavors that Nick and I could not stop eating. It's delicious served with a carrot and pea duo, and rice—a combination of yellow, wild, and white rice. This crowd-pleasing, complementing, and colorful entrée won't disappoint. Tasters might think you're a superstar—my client certainly did. Bonus? It couldn't be simpler. The chicken is cooked before it's added to the sauce, so plan accordingly.

8 servings

2 tablespoons butter
1 teaspoon curry powder
1 cup chopped onion
1 teaspoon cinnamon
½ cup orange marmalade
1 can (28 ounces) chopped tomatoes
1 teaspoon salt
A few grindings of black pepper
1 pound bite-sized pieces of cooked white-meat chicken
1 can (14.1 ounces) hearts of palm, sliced

1. Preheat the oven to 350°F.
2. Melt the butter in a sauté pan over moderate heat. Add the curry powder and stir for about 1 minute. Add the onion and sauté for 5 minutes or until softened. Add the cinnamon, orange marmalade, tomatoes, salt, and pepper. Add the chicken pieces and hearts of palm, and cook until heated through. Serve immediately.

Chicken, Vegetables, and Brown Rice Pasta with Red Curry Coconut Sauce

In this locally and globally charged dish there is an interesting contrast of flavors. The rich and creamy coconut milk combined with fiery red curry paste and the distinct flavor of peanut butter marries well with the assorted vegetables, chicken, and brown rice pasta. Plan accordingly; the chicken is cooked before it is added to the remaining ingredients. Coconut milk naturally separates and hardens—it will become fluid when heated. Shake the can well before opening and stir until fully blended before adding to the onion and mushroom mixture.

4 to 6 servings

1 tablespoon coconut oil
1 cup sliced onions
1 package (8 ounces) or about 8 to 10 medium-sized white mushrooms, sliced
1 can (14 ounces) coconut milk
2 tablespoons red curry paste
2 tablespoons chunky peanut butter
1 teaspoon salt
2 cups cauliflower florets broken into bite-sized pieces
1 cup carrots, julienned
2 cups bite-sized cooked white-meat chicken
1 package (8 ounces) brown rice pasta

1. Fill a large pot with water and bring to a boil.
2. While you're waiting for the water to boil, heat the oil in a large pot over moderate heat. Sauté the onions and mushrooms until tender. Add the coconut milk, red curry paste, peanut butter, and salt. Stir to combine. Allow the mixture to simmer while you cook the vegetables.
3. Fill a large pot with a few inches of water and place a steamer basket on top—the water should be just below the holes of the steamer. Cover the pot and bring the water to a boil. When the water has boiled, steam the cauliflower and carrots for 7 to 10 minutes or until just fork-tender.

4. Add the vegetables and the chicken to the red curry/coconut mixture. Allow it to simmer while you cook the noodles.

5. Cook the pasta in boiling water according to package directions. Drain and divide the pasta among rimmed serving bowls. Spoon the coconut sauce over the pasta. Serve immediately.

MOIST AND DELICIOUS HOLIDAY TURKEY

This turkey recipe is a Dunnington Thanksgiving tradition that has satisfied many a diner at our holiday table. There aren't any measurements for the rub seasoning because you need more or less, depending on the size of the turkey. No place for perfection with this recipe; we wing the ingredient amounts every year and are never disappointed with the outcome. Cheesecloth can be found in the cooking or kitchen supplies aisle of most grocery stores nationwide, online, or in a kitchen supply store. Plan accordingly; the turkey is prepped the day before you cook it.

Olive oil
Worcestershire sauce
Dry mustard
Apple cider vinegar
Salt and pepper
Turkey, neck and giblets removed from the body cavity
1 onion, cut in half
2 stalks of celery, cut in half
A few sprigs of parsley
2 slices of uncooked bacon
1 stick butter, cut into chunks
Natural cotton cheesecloth
Olive oil
2 cups chicken broth

1. In a medium bowl, combine the olive oil, Worcestershire sauce, dry mustard, and a little bit of apple cider vinegar. (The thickness should be similar to prepared mustard.) Season the mixture generously with salt and pepper.
2. Rub the inside and outside of the turkey with the olive oil/Worcestershire mixture. (If you run out of the mixture, make another batch.)
3. Place the onion, celery, and parsley sprigs inside the turkey. Lay 1 slice of bacon across each breast of the turkey.
4. In the little crevice between the drumstick and the body of the turkey, place chunks of butter.
5. Cut enough cheesecloth to cover the turkey. In a large bowl, soak the cheesecloth in the olive oil. Cover the turkey with the olive oil-soaked cheesecloth. Transfer the turkey to a roasting pan large enough to accommodate it. Cover and refrigerate until the following day.

6. Preheat the oven to 300°F.

7. Add the chicken broth to the bottom of the roasting pan. Cook the turkey, uncovered, according to the recommendations at the end of this recipe.

8. Baste the turkey only once or twice during the course of cooking. Allow it to stand for about 30 minutes before removing the cheesecloth and carving. (To remove the cheesecloth, use scissors to cut it and carefully remove it, making certain you don't pull the skin off when removing the cheesecloth.)

COOKING TIMES

7 to 10 pounds, 30 minutes per pound
11 to 15 pounds, 20 minutes per pound
16 to 18 pounds, 18 minutes per pound
19 to 20 pounds, 15 minutes per pound
21 to 23 pounds, 13 minutes per pound

OLD BAY CRAB CAKES

The flavor of crabmeat differs, depending on where it comes from. This leaves cooks to use their own judgment when seasoning. Domestic crabmeat is sweeter and typically has the tasty mustard that gives it a zestier flavor. While both types of crabmeat work to make a crab cake, I prefer domestic over imported for its sweet flavor. If you can only get imported, season the crabmeat with a little more mayonnaise, Old Bay, and Dijon mustard.

4 crab cakes

1 egg
2 slices of bread, crusts removed, torn into small pieces
2 tablespoons mayonnaise
2 teaspoons Old Bay seasoning
1 teaspoon Dijon-style mustard
1 pound backfin crabmeat, picked free of any shell
2 tablespoons butter

1. In a medium bowl, lightly beat the egg. Add the bread pieces and toss the combination with a fork. Allow the bread to absorb the egg for about 5 minutes. Add the mayonnaise, Old Bay seasoning, and mustard. Combine until fully blended. Gently fold in the crabmeat.
2. Form crabmeat mixture into patties.
3. In a large skillet over medium heat, melt the butter. Add the crab cakes, and cook until lightly brown on each side and cooked through. Serve immediately.

HERBED TROUT WITH FRIED CARROTS

Nick dubbed this fantastic-tasting entrée "Invite Friends for Dinner." With so much flavor and texture, it reminds me of so many wonderful fish dishes I've had in high-end restaurants. Any leftover herbed marinade makes for a great-tasting stock for fish soup, stew, or chowder. For a quick, impressive, and balanced meal, serve fish over quinoa, regular or pearl couscous, and a fresh unadorned seasonal vegetable.

4 servings

4 fresh trout fillets
2 cups water
2 vegetable bouillon cubes
4 tablespoons butter
¼ cup fresh parsley, minced
4 teaspoons grated lemon zest
2 teaspoons thyme
2 medium carrots, shredded (using a vegetable peeler)
Neutral oil (expeller-pressed canola, high-oleic safflower, or sunflower oil) for frying carrots

1. Place the fish in a single layer in a rimmed baking dish.
2. Bring two cups of water to a boil. Add the bouillon cubes and stir until they dissolve. Add the butter, parsley, grated lemon zest, and thyme. Stir until the butter has melted.
3. When the seasoned broth has cooled, pour the mixture over the fillets. Allow the fish to marinate at room temperature for about a half hour.
4. Preheat the oven to 350°F.
5. Bake the fish for 12 to 15 minutes or until it flakes easily when tested with a fork.
6. While the fish is baking, prepare the fried carrots. In a large skillet, heat the oil over moderately high heat. Add the carrots and sauté until brown, turning constantly. (Watch closely because there is a narrow margin between brown and crispy carrots and blackened carrots.)
7. Before transferring the fish to serving plates, baste it with the seasoned broth. If desired, carefully remove the skin and place the fillets on serving plates. Top each fillet with carrots. Serve immediately.

CREAMY SHRIMP AND PASTA WITH ARUGULA PESTO

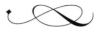

When arugula is brimming in the garden, I often prepare this colorful, impressive, and flavorful meal. I use A.A. Borsari, a citrus seasoning blend made of sea salt, garlic, basil, rosemary, black pepper, lemon peel, and nutmeg. For more about this blend, see seasoning salts in the Product Reference Guide (page 233). A similar blend intended for seafood will work if you can't locate Borsari. We like to serve the pasta with garlic bread or warm, crusty dinner rolls.

4 servings

2 cloves garlic
3 cups arugula (about 3 generous handfuls)
⅓ cup pecorino cheese, grated
½ teaspoon salt
¼ cup olive oil
¼ cup heavy cream
4 cups raw egg noodles
3 tablespoons unbleached all-purpose flour
1½ teaspoons A.A. Bosari Citrus Seasoning Blend
1 pound raw shrimp, peeled, deveined, and patted dry
2 tablespoons neutral oil (expeller-pressed canola, high-oleic safflower, or sunflower oil)

1. Bring a large pot of water to a boil.
2. In a food processor, pulse the garlic a few times. Add the arugula, pecorino cheese, and salt. Pulse until combined. Slowly pour the olive oil through the feed tube, and whirl the mixture until well combined. Transfer the pesto to a medium bowl. Add the cream to the pesto and stir until fully blended. Set aside.
3. Cook the pasta according to the package directions.
4. While the pasta is cooking, combine the flour with the citrus seasoning blend in a small bowl. Dredge the shrimp in the seasoned flour mixture, coating them completely.
5. Cook the shrimp in batches. Heat the oil in a large skillet over medium heat. Add a batch of shrimp and cook for 2 to 3 minutes, or until light brown on both sides. Repeat until all the shrimp are cooked.
6. Drain the pasta. Return the pasta to the pot and add the creamy pesto to the pasta and toss until well combined. Add the shrimp to the pesto/pasta. Warm the combination over a low heat, stirring constantly. Serve immediately.

LEMON-MARINATED CATFISH WITH ARTICHOKE HEARTS AND KALAMATA OLIVES

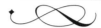

Brimming with flavor, this entrée is simple to assemble, elegant with an impressive presentation. The flavor of the catfish speaks for itself, so the side dishes don't need to be overly embellished.

4 servings

16 thinly sliced lemons (about 2 to 3 lemons), seeds removed
4 fresh catfish fillets
½ cup extra-virgin olive oil
Salt
A few grindings of black pepper
1 can (14 ounces) water-packed artichoke hearts, drained and quartered
½ cup Kalamata olives, pitted and roughly chopped
Freshly minced parsley (garnish)

1. Preheat the oven to 350°F.
2. Arrange 8 of the lemon slices in the bottom of a 15 x 10 x 2-inch baking dish and top with the catfish fillets. Top the catfish with the remaining slices. Pour the olive oil evenly over the fillets, and season with salt and pepper.
3. Bake the fillets, uncovered, for 20 minutes.
4. Remove the lemon slices from the top of the fillets. Distribute the artichoke hearts and olives over the fillets. Spoon olive oil essence over the combination.
5. Bake for an additional 10 minutes.
6. Carefully transfer the fillets, without the bottom layer of lemon slices, to individual serving plates. Garnish with parsley. Serve immediately.

Apricot Tomatoes with Hearts of Palm, Shrimp, and Feta

This is a household favorite, and with good reason: It's soothing and infused with a myriad of flavors. Don't limit the protein part of the dish to shrimp. I've made it using cooked meatballs, shredded cooked chicken breast, and firm white fish like cod, haddock, and halibut. Any one of these options works in this lively tomato-based meal. This dish is also delicious spooned over tortellini; the savory tomatoes and sweet apricots, the briny olives, and capers are delicious contrasts to cheese-filled tortellini. Huzzah!

8 servings

2 cans (28 ounces each) diced tomatoes
1 cup dried apricots, chopped
½ cup Spanish olives, chopped
¼ cup capers
¼ cup olive oil
8 large garlic cloves, chopped
2 tablespoons granulated sugar
2 tablespoons oregano
2 bay leaves
1 teaspoon salt
Several grindings of black pepper
1 can (14 ounces) hearts of palm, drained and sliced
1 pound cooked shrimp
1 cup feta cheese (or desired amount), crumbled
Cooked tortellini, if desired

1. Combine the tomatoes with the apricots, olives, capers, olive oil, garlic, sugar, oregano, bay leaves, salt, and pepper in a large pot. Gently bring the mixture to a boil. Reduce the heat, cover, and simmer for about 1 hour.
2. Add the hearts of palm and shrimp. Warm the mixture until heated through. Remove the bay leaves. Serve immediately, and pass the feta cheese to your guests.

BAKED COD WITH TOASTED COCONUT AND PINEAPPLE SALSA

This beautiful array of fresh, colorful, and tasty ingredients makes the perfect topping for a mild white fish. Our favorite is cod. I toast the coconut in the toaster oven set at 350°. Watch closely; it doesn't take long before it's chestnut brown in spots. For optimum flavor, the pineapple should be ripe. I use jarred roasted red bell peppers found in the condiment aisle of the grocery store. You can prepare the salsa in advance and add the avocado just before serving.

8 servings

8 pieces cod fillets
Olive oil
2 cups fresh pineapple, chopped
½ cup roasted red bell peppers, chopped
½ cup shredded carrots
¼ cup shredded sweetened coconut, toasted
¼ cup macadamia nuts, chopped and toasted
¼ cup scallions (green onions), sliced
Salt, to taste
1 ripe avocado, cut into bite-sized pieces

1. Preheat the oven to 400°F.
2. Place the cod fillets on a rimmed baking sheet lined with parchment paper. Drizzle them with olive oil. Bake for 10 to 12 minutes or until the fish just begins to flake.
3. In a medium bowl, combine the pineapple with the chopped red bell peppers, shredded carrots, toasted coconut, macadamia nuts, and scallions. Drizzle the mixture with olive oil and season with salt. Just before serving, add the avocado, and gently stir just to combine.
4. Serve immediately, and pass the pineapple salsa to your guests.

Quinoa Cheeseburgers with Curried Cucumber Yogurt Sauce

Here is a celebration of flavors and textures that was developed from having leftover chickpeas and quinoa. I initially served the flavorful burgers on yellow-corn taco shells because that is what I had on hand (the crispy shells add another dimension of texture) and never converted to the traditional burger roll. If you're sensitive to spicy, you can reduce the amount of red curry paste. Cheddar cheese can be used in place of habanero (hot pepper) cheddar.

4 burgers

CURRIED CUCUMBER YOGURT SAUCE

½ teaspoon red curry paste (or ¼ teaspoon if you're sensitive to spicy)
¾ cup plain yogurt
¼ cup sour cream
1 cup cucumber, peeled, seeds removed, and shredded
¼ cup scallions (green onions), minced
⅛ cup shredded sweetened coconut
½ teaspoon salt

1. Combine the red curry paste with the yogurt and sour cream in a medium bowl. Add the cucumber, ¼ cup scallions, coconut, and salt. Combine until well blended. Cover and refrigerate until serving time.

QUINOA CHEESEBURGERS

½ cup water
⅓ cup plain quinoa
1 teaspoon red curry paste
½ teaspoon salt
1 egg
1 cup chickpeas
2 cloves garlic, minced
1 cup cooked quinoa

75

1 cup habanero cheddar cheese, shredded
⅛ cup scallions (green onions), thinly sliced
1 tablespoon coconut oil
4 taco shells, cooked according to package directions
Shredded lettuce or microgreens

1. Bring the water to a boil in a small pan. Stir in the quinoa, remove from heat, cover, and let the quinoa stand for 5 minutes. Set aside.
2. Combine the red curry paste with the salt and egg in a medium bowl and beat until well blended. Roughly mash the chickpeas. (I use a potato masher.) Add the mashed chickpeas, garlic, cooked quinoa, cheese, and scallions to the egg mixture, and stir the ingredients until incorporated.
3. Divide the mixture into four portions and shape into patties.
4. Heat the oil in a large skillet over medium heat. Add the patties and cook until light brown on each side and heated through. Place the burgers on top of the taco shells. Pass the curried cucumber yogurt sauce and shredded lettuce or microgreens to your guests.

CHEESY EGGPLANT, BEAN, AND VEGETABLE CASSEROLE

This vegetarian, weeknight-friendly meal is teeming with color, flavor, and a delightful variety of textures. Serve with cast-iron honey-glazed cornbread (page 115), Russian black bread, or hearty whole wheat.

8 servings

1 medium eggplant, cut into ½-inch slices
Olive oil
Coarse salt
1 tablespoon neutral oil (expeller-pressed canola, high-oleic safflower, or sunflower oil)
1 cup chopped onion
4 cloves garlic, sliced
1½ teaspoons cumin
2 teaspoons oregano
1 can (28 ounces) fire-roasted tomatoes
¼ cup fresh parsley, minced
1 cup carrots, julienned
1 cup cooked corn kernels
1 can (14 ounces) white kidney beans, drained
½ cup fresh grated Asiago cheese
1 cup shredded mozzarella cheese

1. Preheat the oven to 350°F.
2. Place the eggplant slices on a parchment-lined rimmed baking sheet and brush them with olive oil. Season with coarse salt and cook for a half hour or until tender. When the eggplant is cool enough to handle, cut into cubes. Set aside.
3. Heat the oil in a large pot over moderate heat and sauté the onions until tender. Add the garlic and cook for a few minutes. Add the cumin and oregano and cook for about 1 minute. Add the tomatoes, parsley, and carrots. Cover the pot, and increase the heat and cook for 5 to 10 minutes or until the carrots are tender. Add the corn kernels and beans, and stir to combine.
4. Spread half of the tomato mixture in the bottom of an 11 x 7 x 2-inch baking dish. Top the tomatoes with the cubed eggplant and ¼ cup of Asiago cheese. Top the cheese with the remaining tomato mixture, mozzarella cheese, and the remaining ¼ cup of Asiago cheese. Cover and cook for 30 minutes or until bubbly. Remove cover and cook for an additional 10 to 15 minutes. Serve immediately.

CREAMY LEMON PENNE PASTA WITH BROCCOLI

Creamy comfort food. Cook the broccoli according to your liking. Keep in mind that broccoli cooks a wee bit longer after it's been steamed, so I prefer to cook it until it's not yet fork-tender.

4 servings

2½ cups broccoli, cut into small bite-sized pieces
3 cups penne pasta
2 tablespoons butter
2 teaspoons grated lemon zest
3 tablespoons fresh lemon juice
¼ teaspoon salt
2 eggs
1 cup milk

1. Fill a large pot with water and bring to a boil. Salt the water if desired.
2. Fill a large pot with a few inches of water and place a steamer basket on top—the water should be just below the holes of the steamer. Cover the pot and bring the water to a boil. When the water has boiled, steam the broccoli until it's not yet fork-tender, 7 to 10 minutes. Transfer the broccoli to a platter and set aside.
3. Cook the pasta in the boiling water according to the package directions. Drain the pasta and add the broccoli. Cover the pot.
4. In a medium skillet over moderate heat, melt the butter. Add the lemon zest, lemon juice, and salt, and cook for 1 minute. Toss the mixture with the pasta and broccoli.
5. In a small bowl, whisk the eggs with the milk until well combined. Add the mixture to the pasta/broccoli mixture and cook over low heat, stirring constantly, for 3 to 4 minutes, or until the mixture thickens slightly. Serve immediately.

HERBED CABBAGE AND MUSHROOM PIE

This recipe from my sister defines hearty vegetarian cozy-up food—the perfect meal to serve on a cold, wintry night.

6 to 8 servings

1¼ cups unbleached all-purpose flour
1 teaspoon salt
8 ounces (block-style) ⅓ less fat cream cheese, divided in half, at room temperature
3 tablespoons butter, softened
4 tablespoons water
5 eggs
1 tablespoon neutral oil (expeller-pressed canola, high-oleic safflower, or sunflower oil)
6 cups savoy cabbage, shredded
1 package (8 ounces) or about 6 to 8 medium-sized white mushrooms, sliced
1 cup onion, sliced
1 teaspoon basil
1 teaspoon marjoram
1 teaspoon tarragon
½ teaspoon salt
A few grindings of black pepper

1. Combine the flour and salt in a medium bowl. Add the cream cheese and butter and, using your fingers, mix until well combined. Add the water to create a smooth dough—you may need to add more water. Divide the dough into thirds, reserving one-third for the top crust and the rest for the bottom crust. Cover the dough pieces and chill for about a half hour.
2. Fill a medium pot three-quarters full with water and bring to a boil. Add the eggs, reduce the heat slightly (water should be actively rumbling), and cook the eggs uncovered for 15 minutes. Drain and peel them. Set aside. When the eggs are cool enough to handle, chop them.
3. Roll out the bottom crust portion of the pie shell. Transfer to a 9-inch pie plate. Flute the edges. Set aside.

4. Heat the oil in a large skillet over moderate heat. Add the cabbage, mushrooms, and onions. Cook, stirring frequently, for 8 to 10 minutes. Remove from heat and season the mixture with basil, marjoram, tarragon, salt, and pepper.

5. Preheat the oven to 400°F.

6. Spread 4 ounces of cream cheese over the bottom of the pie crust. Top with the chopped eggs. Top the eggs with the herbed cabbage mixture.

7. Roll out the remaining crust and place it over the cabbage. Press the edges of the top crust with the edges of the bottom crust. Cut a few short slashes through the top crust.

8. Bake at 400°F for 15 minutes. Reduce the oven temperature to 350°F and bake for an additional 25 minutes. Serve immediately.

PALAK PANEER

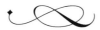

If you're not familiar with this delicious Indian dish, palak is the creamy spinach part of this simple vegetarian dish. The spinach is combined with robust flavored spices and milk, and blended until it has a smooth consistency. Paneer is a fresh, unsalted, white, non-melting cheese with a mild, milky flavor, similar to mozzarella, but not soft. When paneer is sautéed, as it is in this recipe, it brings out the flavor of this delectable cheese. The combination is a flavor sensation with a wonderful combination of textures. Paneer is available in most grocery stores nationwide.

4 to 6 servings

3 tablespoons neutral oil (expeller-pressed canola, high-oleic safflower, or
*   sunflower oil)*
1 teaspoon ground cumin
1 teaspoon turmeric
½ teaspoon ground ginger
2 tablespoons red curry paste
16 ounces frozen chopped spinach, defrosted, drained, and squeezed dry
2 tablespoons flour
2 cups milk
1 teaspoon salt
8 ounces paneer cheese, cut into bite-sized pieces

1. Heat 2 tablespoons of oil in a large pot over moderate heat. Add the cumin, turmeric, and ginger. Stir until well combined. Cook for about 1 minute or until fragrant. Add the red curry paste and spinach, and stir until the ingredients are incorporated. Add the flour and stir until it's combined with the spinach mixture. Slowly add the milk, stirring constantly. Add the salt, reduce the heat, and simmer for 5 to 7 minutes.

2. Transfer the mixture to a food processor and purée until smooth. Return the mixture to the pot to keep warm while you prepare the paneer.

3. In a sauté pan, heat 1 tablespoon of oil over moderately high heat and sauté the paneer until golden brown.

4. Spoon palak into shallow-rimmed bowls. Top palak with paneer, distributing equally. Serve immediately.

WILD PORCINI MUSHROOM LASAGNA

My good friend David Frank is as passionate about food as he is about letting friends in on anything new and different. When he shared his latest find, Exclusivo Wild Porcini Sauce, he said, "This is the best sauce I've ever tasted. Let me know what you think." Based on the sauce's ingredients (eggplant, tomatoes, onions, garlic, olive oil, wild porcini mushrooms, celery, carrots, and several seasonings)—not to mention my respect for David's impeccable palate—I knew I wanted to taste-test. This sauce is ambrosial, and this lasagna is one you will not soon forget. Most Italian grocery stores carry the sauce, or you can purchase it online—buying in quantity is encouraged. This can be prepared in advance, covered, and refrigerated; just allow enough time for the lasagna to come to room temperature before cooking.

8 servings

2 eggs
2 containers (15 ounces each) ricotta cheese
1 pound fresh mozzarella cheese, shredded
½ cup fresh grated Parmesan cheese
½ cup fresh parsley, minced
1 teaspoon salt
Several grindings of black pepper
1 (31 ounce) jar Wild Porcini Sauce (stir before using)
9 no-boil (or oven-ready) lasagna noodles

1. Preheat the oven to 350°F.
2. In a large bowl, lightly beat the eggs. Add the ricotta cheese, half of the mozzarella cheese, ¼ cup of the Parmesan cheese, parsley, salt, and pepper. Mix until fully combined.
3. Spoon about 1¼ cups of the sauce into a 13 x 9 x 2-inch baking dish. Top it with 3 lasagna noodles in a single layer. Spread about a third of the ricotta mixture over the noodles. Top the ricotta with about 1¼ cups of the sauce and top the sauce with 3 noodles and another layer of the ricotta mixture (about half the remaining amount).
4. Top the ricotta mixture with the remaining 3 noodles, the remaining ricotta mixture, and the remaining mozzarella cheese. Sprinkle the remaining Parmesan cheese over the mozzarella and top with the remaining sauce.
5. Cover and bake for 45 minutes. Remove the cover and bake for an additional 15 minutes. Let the lasagna rest for about 15 minutes before serving.

Vegetarian Side Dishes

SALADS, SIDE DISHES, AND POTATOES

Side dishes took center stage on our plates because my mother made sure to bring out their flavor through the use of seasonings and creative food pairings. For me, a meal isn't complete without complementary side dishes. In this chapter are crowd-pleasing vegetarian dishes that can stand alone as a main dish or be paired with an entrée.

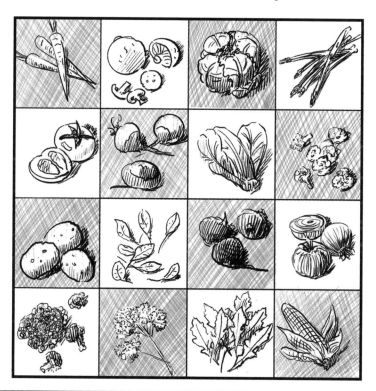

RECIPE INDEX

SALADS

Arugula, Mango, and Hearts of Palm Salad with Salty Lime Dressing 85
Wild Rice Salad with Cherries and Feta 86
Hearty Cabbage and Vegetable Salad with Celery Seed Dressing 87
Golden Beet, Arugula, Pomegranate, and Feta Salad with Blood Orange Dressing 88
Heirloom Tomato and Mozzarella Salad with Toasted Pesto Crumbs 89
Asparagus and Strawberry Salad with Grilled Halloumi 90-91
Quintessential Caesar Salad 92

SIDE DISHES

Asparagus with Crispy-Fried Shallots and Brown Butter Bread Crumbs 93
Curried Cauliflower with Toasted Pecans 94
Spinach-Stuffed Puff Pastry 95
Sesame-Roasted Broccoli 96
Marinated Cauliflower 97
Curry Cumin Coconut Cauliflower with Prunes and Peanuts 98
Honey-Buttered Peppered Turnips and Sweet Peas 99
Gingered Tomatoes with Cinnamon 100

POTATOES

Buttery Buttermilk Parmesan-Stuffed Potatoes 101
New Potatoes with Shitake Mushrooms and Brie 102
Roasted Potatoes with Minted Garlic 103
Simple Creamy Potatoes 104
Roasted Curried Potatoes 105

ARUGULA, MANGO, AND HEARTS OF PALM SALAD WITH SALTY LIME DRESSING

In this locally and globally charged salad, I've combined arugula, red cabbage, fiber-rich hearts of palm, sweet mango, coconut, crunchy macadamia nuts, and black sesame seeds for a lively contrast of colors and textures. The salty lime dressing is the perfect complement to this salad and its many tropical ingredients. For the best flavor results, the mango should be ripe.

6 servings

⅓ cup olive oil
¼ cup fresh lime juice
1 teaspoon salt
6 very generous handfuls of arugula
1 cup thinly shredded red cabbage
1 ripe mango, cut into bite-sized pieces
1 can (14 ounces) hearts of palm, drained and sliced
½ cup macadamia nuts, roasted
Shredded sweetened coconut
Black sesame seeds

1. Combine the olive oil with the lime juice and salt in a 1-cup jar with a tight-fitting lid. Shake until well blended. Set aside.
2. Place the arugula and red cabbage in a large bowl. Give the dressing a good shake and toss the leaves with enough dressing to coat them. Divide the lettuce among 6 serving plates.
3. In a small bowl, combine the mango, hearts of palm, and macadamia nuts. Toss with enough dressing to coat the ingredients. Top the arugula and red cabbage with the mango mixture, distributing ingredients evenly. Sprinkle with shredded coconut and black sesame seeds. Serve immediately.

WILD RICE SALAD WITH CHERRIES AND FETA

When the outside temperatures start inching down, I often serve this hearty, colorful, and complementary combination. Plan accordingly; the wild rice takes about 45 minutes to cook (or more, depending on the brand) and has to cool before it's added to the remaining ingredients.

6 to 8 servings

1 cup wild rice
¼ cup apple cider vinegar
1 teaspoon salt
Several grindings of black pepper
1 teaspoon Dijon-style mustard
¾ cup extra-virgin olive oil
½ cup shredded carrots
½ cup celery, sliced
¼ cup fresh parsley, minced
½ cup dried cherries
½ cup crumbled feta cheese
¼ cup slivered almonds, toasted

1. Cook the wild rice according to the package directions. Once cooked, transfer the rice to a large serving bowl and allow it to cool completely.
2. Combine the apple cider vinegar, salt, pepper, and mustard in a 2-cup jar with a tight-fitting lid. Shake until the ingredients are well blended and the salt has dissolved. Add the olive oil and shake again to combine the ingredients. Store the vinaigrette dressing at room temperature until ready to serve.
3. Toss the rice with the carrots, celery, parsley, and cherries. Shake the dressing well and toss the rice mixture with just enough dressing to coat the ingredients. Transfer the mixture to a rimmed serving platter and top with feta and slivered almonds. Serve immediately. Refrigerate any unused portion of vinaigrette dressing.

HEARTY CABBAGE AND VEGETABLE SALAD WITH CELERY SEED DRESSING

Chock full of color and nutrient-rich raw ingredients, this salad promises to please. You will have more celery seed dressing than what is needed in this recipe. However, it is delicious tossed with just about any fresh leafy greens or vegetables, and it keeps for several weeks in the refrigerator.

6 servings

⅓ cup granulated sugar
1 teaspoon salt
1 teaspoon dry mustard
1 teaspoon freshly minced onion
¼ cup apple cider vinegar
1 cup canola oil
1 teaspoon celery seeds
5 cups red cabbage, shredded
1 cup carrots, julienned
1 cup celery, sliced
½ cup frozen peas, thawed
1 cup feta cheese, crumbled
½ cup toasted sunflower seeds

1. In a medium bowl or the bowl of a stand mixer, combine the sugar, salt, and dry mustard. Add the onion and apple cider vinegar and combine until the sugar has dissolved. Slowly add the oil and whisk until the dressing thickens. Add the celery seeds and whisk until fully blended. Transfer the mixture to a 2-cup jar with a tight-fitting lid. Set aside.
2. In a large bowl, combine the cabbage, carrots, celery, and peas. Shake the dressing and toss the salad with enough dressing to coat the vegetables. Divide the salad among 6 salad dishes, and top with feta and sunflower seeds. Serve immediately.

GOLDEN BEET, ARUGULA, POMEGRANATE, AND FETA SALAD WITH BLOOD ORANGE DRESSING

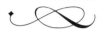

For a unique presentation, I like to serve this beautiful cold-weather salad in savoy cabbage leaves. If you don't want to serve it this way, serve just as you would any other salad. Extra dressing will keep for several days in the refrigerator and can be tossed with other leafy greens. If you can't get blood orange juice, regular orange juice can be substituted with the same results.

Serves 6

4 medium golden beets, quartered
1 teaspoon salt
1 teaspoon Dijon-style mustard
Several grindings of black pepper
¼ cup blood orange juice, freshly squeezed
¾ cup expeller-pressed organic canola oil
6 generous handfuls of baby arugula
6 savoy cabbage leaves, if desired
½ cup pomegranate seeds
½ cup feta cheese, crumbled
¼ cup toasted sunflower seeds
Microgreens (garnish)

1. Bring a large pot of water to a boil. Cook the beets for 15 to 20 minutes or until fork-tender, depending on size. When the beets are cool enough to handle, pinch off the skin.
2. Julienne-cut the beets and place them in a medium bowl.
3. Combine the salt, Dijon mustard, pepper, and blood orange juice in a 2-cup jar with a tight-fitting lid. Shake the mixture vigorously. Add the oil and shake well.
4. Lightly coat the beets with the dressing.
5. Toss the arugula with enough dressing to coat the leaves. Place savoy cabbage leaves on serving plates and top them with arugula, distributing evenly. Top each with the beets, pomegranate seeds, feta, and sunflower seeds. Garnish with microgreens. Serve immediately.

HEIRLOOM TOMATO AND MOZZARELLA SALAD WITH TOASTED PESTO CRUMBS

When tomato plants are at their peak of munificence, I prepare this super-simple, summer-inspired dish throughout the duration of the tomato season. For a stunning presentation, I love to use a variety of colorful heirloom tomatoes like red, Yellow Boy, orange, and Green Zebra tomatoes with the mozzarella slices. For optimum flavor, a handmade mozzarella is recommended. Plan accordingly; this recipe calls for toasted pesto crumbs (see page 149).

4 servings

8 slices of a variety of heirloom tomatoes
8 slices fresh mozzarella cheese
Toasted pesto crumbs

1. Arrange tomato slices alternately with mozzarella slices on each plate. Generously top with pesto crumbs. Serve immediately.

ASPARAGUS AND STRAWBERRY SALAD WITH GRILLED HALLOUMI

When these farm stars come into season at the same time, I love combining the savory and slender green stalks with juicy sweet strawberries. This tasty and colorful representation of the late-springtime harvest contrasts beautifully with halloumi cheese. Informative preparation tips about asparagus can be found in the Product Reference Guide (page 233). Extra dressing complements just about any tossed salad. Strawberries and asparagus are both best eaten the day you purchase and/or harvest them. This salad is not a good keeper; consume it the day you serve it.

8 servings

1 teaspoon salt
Several grindings of black pepper
1 teaspoon Dijon mustard
¼ cup apple cider vinegar
¾ cup extra-virgin olive oil
1 bunch fresh asparagus spears, washed, tough ends removed
1 pint strawberries, capped and quartered
Neutral oil (expeller-pressed canola, high-oleic safflower, or sunflower oil)
1 package (8.8 ounces) halloumi cheese, sliced
Microgreens (garnish)

1. In a 2-cup jar with a tight-fitting lid, combine the salt, pepper, mustard, and apple cider vinegar. Shake until the ingredients are well blended and the salt has dissolved. Add the olive oil and shake again to combine the ingredients. Store at room temperature until ready to serve. Shake well just prior to using.
2. Bring a large pot of water to a boil. Cook the asparagus in the boiling water until just fork-tender, about 5 minutes for medium-sized spears. (Check every minute or so by piercing the spears with a sharp knife.) Once cooked, immediately submerge the spears in an ice water bath. When cool, drain, pat dry, and cut into 1-inch pieces. Set aside.
3. In a medium bowl, combine the asparagus with the strawberries.
4. In a large skillet, heat the oil over moderate heat and cook the halloumi slices on each side until brown in spots.

5. Transfer the cheese slices to serving plates.

6. Toss the asparagus and strawberries with just enough dressing to coat the ingredients. (Refrigerate any unused dressing.) Top each halloumi slice with the asparagus and strawberry mixture, distributing evenly. Top each with a garnish of microgreens if desired. Serve immediately.

QUINTESSENTIAL CAESAR SALAD

Italian immigrant Caesar Cardini presumably tossed the first Caesar salad in July 1924 when he was running low on food and assembled a salad for his guests from what was left over in the kitchen. A familiar-sounding scenario. Here is my version of the classic Caesar—sans the raw egg. For the cheese, I use pecorino pepato, an intense, salty sheep's milk cheese studded with peppercorns. I think it's the perfect cheese for a Caesar salad. Pecorino pepato can typically be found near the Parmesan in the specialty cheese section. Leftover dressing will keep for several days refrigerated.

6 servings

2 cups French bread, cut into bite-sized cubes
Olive oil
Garlic powder
2 tablespoons red wine vinegar
2 teaspoons Dijon-style mustard
2 teaspoons Worcestershire sauce
1 clove garlic, minced
1 teaspoon anchovy paste
½ teaspoon salt
Several grindings of black pepper
½ cup mayonnaise
6 generous handfuls of romaine lettuce, torn into bite-sized pieces
⅓ cup fresh pecorino pepato cheese, shredded
Anchovy fillets (optional)

1. Preheat the oven to 400°F.
2. Toss the French bread cubes with the olive oil and generously season them with garlic powder. Transfer the cubes to a rimmed baking sheet, arrange in a single layer (a good shake does the trick), and bake for about 15 minutes or until toasty brown.
3. In a medium bowl, combine the red wine vinegar, mustard, Worcestershire sauce, garlic, anchovy paste, salt, and black pepper. Whisk until the ingredients are evenly distributed. Add the mayonnaise and whisk until fully incorporated.
4. Place the romaine leaves in a large bowl and toss with just enough dressing to coat the leaves.
5. Transfer the dressed leaves to serving plates, and top each with cheese and croutons. Garnish with anchovy fillets if desired. Serve immediately.

ASPARAGUS WITH CRISPY-FRIED SHALLOTS AND BROWN BUTTER BREAD CRUMBS

This asparagus dish, with its complementing contrasts of textures, is a lovely springtime side dish to serve with beef, lamb, fish, or chicken. Informative preparation tips about asparagus can be found in the Product Reference Guide (page 233).

4 servings

2 tablespoons butter
¼ cup shallots, thinly sliced
¼ cup dry bread crumbs
1 bunch asparagus spears, washed, tough ends removed

1. Bring a large pot of water to a boil. Cook the asparagus in the boiling water until just fork-tender, about 5 minutes for medium-sized spears. (Check every minute or so by piercing the spears with a sharp knife.) Once cooked, immediately submerge the spears in an ice water bath. When cool, drain and keep them at room temperature until serving time.

2. Melt the butter in a medium skillet over moderate heat and sauté the shallots until tender. Add the bread crumbs and cook, stirring constantly, until they are chestnut brown. Set aside.

3. Just prior to serving, heat the asparagus by pouring boiling water over the spears. Drain them and place on a kitchen towel to absorb any excess water. Transfer the asparagus to a platter and top them with the shallot/brown butter bread crumb mixture. Serve immediately.

CURRIED CAULIFLOWER WITH TOASTED PECANS

This complementary combination has a creamy yet crunchy texture, with the perfect hint of sweet and savory spices that defines the flavor of curry. You can cook the cauliflower and prepare the curried mayonnaise in advance. It's best, however, to toss the cauliflower and top it with the pecans just prior to serving.

10 to 12 servings

1 medium head of cauliflower, broken into uniform, bite-sized pieces
1 cup mayonnaise
1 teaspoon curry powder
¼ cup fresh minced parsley
1 cup chopped pecans, toasted

1. Fill a large pot with a few inches of water and place a steamer basket on top—the water should be just below the holes of the steamer. Cover the pot and bring the water to a boil. When the water has boiled, steam the cauliflower for 7 to 10 minutes or until just fork-tender.
2. Transfer the cauliflower to a serving platter and allow the cauliflower to cool completely.
3. In a large bowl, combine the mayonnaise, curry powder, and parsley. Add the cooled cauliflower to the mixture and combine, evenly distributing the ingredients. Top the cauliflower with pecans. Serve immediately.

SPINACH-STUFFED PUFF PASTRY

This simple, elegant, and impressive-looking side dish complements chicken, seafood, lamb, and beef. I especially love to serve it for Christmas dinner with roast beef, beef tenderloin, or a standing rib roast. Puff pastry needs to thaw before it's ready to roll. Not every brand has the same thawing directions; check the package before you make this recipe.

12 servings

2 tablespoons butter
1 cup onion, chopped
2 cloves garlic, minced
16 ounces frozen chopped spinach, defrosted, drained, and squeezed dry
1 container (8 ounces) mascarpone cheese
1 teaspoon salt
Several grindings of black pepper
⅛ teaspoon nutmeg
2 sheets puff pastry dough, thawed
1 egg, lightly beaten

1. In a large skillet over moderate heat, melt the butter and sauté the onion until translucent. Add the garlic and cook for a few minutes. Remove from heat and add the spinach, mascarpone, salt, pepper, and nutmeg. Stir until well combined. Set aside.
2. Preheat the oven to 400°F.
3. Line a rimmed baking sheet with parchment paper.
4. Lightly coat a work surface with flour. Unfold the pastry sheets and roll each one until it is slightly bigger than the original size. Spread half the spinach mixture over the surface of the sheets. Gently roll each one and carefully transfer them to the prepared baking sheet. Brush the top of both rolls with the beaten egg.
5. Bake for 25 minutes or until golden brown. Allow the rolls to cool for about 5 minutes before slicing. Slice each roll into 6 slices. Serve immediately.

SESAME-ROASTED BROCCOLI

This zesty, flavorful broccoli dish is one you will not soon forget.

4 servings

2 tablespoons olive oil
1 tablespoon soy sauce or tamari
1 tablespoon toasted sesame oil
1 tablespoon sesame seeds
½ teaspoon salt
4 cups broccoli florets, broken into bite-sized pieces

1. Preheat the oven to 450°F.
2. Line a rimmed baking sheet with parchment paper.
3. In a large bowl, combine the olive oil, soy sauce or tamari, sesame oil, sesame seeds, and salt. Whisk until well blended. Add the broccoli and toss well.
4. Transfer the broccoli to the prepared baking sheet and bake for 10 minutes or until fork-tender, or to your desired tenderness. Serve immediately.

MARINATED CAULIFLOWER

When cauliflower is in season, I can't seem to get enough of this mellow-tasting, nutritious vegetable. I love to use a combination of purple, golden-yellow, and white cauliflower; the trio turns out a dish that is as tasty as it is beautiful. If you don't want to buy three heads, any one of the colors works with the same flavor results—no matter the color, they all taste the same. The key to the success of this recipe is to combine the vegetable bouillon cube/olive oil mixture with the cauliflower while it's still warm.

4 servings

1 vegetable bouillon cube
¼ cup olive oil
4 cups cauliflower florets broken into bite-sized pieces

1. In a medium bowl, mash the bouillon cube and olive oil with a fork. Blend the mixture until the cube is fully incorporated with the olive oil. Set aside.
2. Fill a large pot with a few inches of water, and place a steamer basket on top. The water should be just below the holes of the steamer. Cover the pot and bring the water to a boil. When the water has boiled, steam the cauliflower for 7 to 10 minutes or just until fork-tender.
3. Immediately transfer the hot cauliflower to the bouillon cube/olive oil mixture and toss to distribute the ingredients evenly. Serve immediately.

Curry Cumin Coconut Cauliflower with Prunes and Peanuts

We usually finish eating this flavor-charged dish alone in one sitting—it's that good. It complements baked chicken in a way you won't forget. Coconut milk naturally separates and hardens; it will become fluid when heated. Shake the can well before opening and stir until fully blended before adding to the cauliflower/onion mixture.

4 to 6 servings

2 tablespoons olive oil
2 teaspoons curry powder
2 teaspoons ground cumin
1 cup sliced onion
6 cups cauliflower, broken into uniform bite-sized pieces
1 can (14 ounces) coconut milk
½ cup chopped prunes
1 teaspoon salt
½ cup roasted and salted peanuts

1. In a large pan over moderate heat, heat the olive oil and add the curry powder and cumin. Cook for about a minute or until fragrant. Add the sliced onion and cauliflower. Stir until the curry and cumin adhere to the cauliflower and onion. Add the coconut milk, prunes, and salt, and stir to combine.
2. Cover and cook the cauliflower for 10 to 15 minutes or until fork-tender—check after 10 minutes. Transfer to a serving bowl and top the cauliflower mixture with peanuts. Serve immediately.

HONEY-BUTTERED PEPPERED TURNIPS AND SWEET PEAS

My mother first served these delicious turnips at an autumn family gathering. She was pleased they received so many oohs and ahhs because she was hesitant to prepare them at all. After all, not everyone is a fan of turnips. One bite, and we were turnip lovers! When buying, look for smaller turnips because they tend to be sweeter than larger ones.

8 servings

4 tablespoons butter
4 tablespoons honey
2 pound turnips, peeled and cut into bite-sized cubes
Several grindings of black pepper
1 cup frozen sweet peas, thawed

1. In a medium saucepan over moderate heat, melt the butter and honey. Add the turnips and several grindings of pepper. Stir to coat the cubes with the butter/honey mixture.
2. Cover, reduce the heat to simmer, and cook the turnips for 12 to 15 minutes or until fork-tender. Stir once or twice during the cooking time. Add the thawed peas and stir to combine. Serve immediately.

GINGERED TOMATOES WITH CINNAMON

This is a popular tomato dish that you can rely on to serve for everyday eating or entertaining, and it pairs beautifully with chicken, beef, and seafood. If you need a brand of ginger preserves, see the Product Reference Guide (page 233).

6 servings

2 tablespoons butter
1 cup chopped onion
1 teaspoon ground cinnamon
½ cup ginger preserves
1 can (28 ounces) diced tomatoes
1 teaspoon salt
Several grindings of black pepper

1. In a medium pan over moderate heat, melt the butter and add the onion. Sauté for about 5 minutes or until tender. Add the cinnamon and stir for about a minute or until fragrant. Add the ginger preserves, tomatoes, salt, and pepper. Bring the mixture to a gentle boil, reduce the heat, and simmer for about 15 minutes. Serve immediately.

BUTTERY BUTTERMILK PARMESAN-STUFFED POTATOES

Because potatoes vary so much in size, you may have to adjust the seasonings to get that creamy consistency and tasty flavor. So add a little more of everything until the flavors hit that perfect comfort-food note. The potatoes can be cooked and stuffed in advance. If you make them in advance, allow them to come to room temperature before reheating.

8 servings

4 medium baking potatoes
½ cup buttermilk
½ cup scallions (green onions), sliced thinly, more for garnish if desired
4 tablespoons butter (¼ cup), softened
½ cup freshly grated Parmesan cheese
Salt and pepper, to taste
Paprika

1. Preheat the oven to 400°F.
2. Bake the potatoes for 45 minutes to 1 hour or until fork-tender.
3. When the potatoes are cool enough to handle, cut them in half and scoop the pulp into a medium bowl or stand mixer. Set the shells aside on a parchment-lined rimmed baking sheet. Add the buttermilk, scallions, butter, Parmesan cheese, salt, and pepper to the potatoes in the bowl. Mix until well blended and creamy. Taste, and adjust the ingredients if necessary. Evenly divide the potato mixture into the shells.
4. Preheat the oven to 350°F.
5. Bake the stuffed potatoes for about 20 minutes or until heated through.
6. Adjust the oven rack to the highest rung, and set the oven temperature to broil. Brown the top of the potatoes. Sprinkle with paprika and garnish with chopped scallions if desired. Serve immediately.

New Potatoes with Shitake Mushrooms and Brie

This company-worthy, rich-tasting, flavorful dish is delicious served with baked chicken or various cuts of beef like tenderloin, roast, or steak. Brie will cut more easily if you place it in the freezer for about 5 minutes. To keep the Brie from sticking to the knife when cutting, coat the knife with butter.

6 servings

1½ pounds medium new potatoes, unpeeled and shredded
2 packages (3.5 ounces each) or 2 cups shitake mushrooms, stems removed, chopped
½ pound Brie, outer rind removed, cubed
1 cup cream
2 cloves garlic, minced
1 teaspoon dried thyme
1½ teaspoons salt
Several grindings of black pepper
3 tablespoons freshly grated Parmesan cheese
½ cup dry bread crumbs

1. Preheat the oven to 350°F.
2. Lightly coat an 11 x 7 x 2-inch baking dish with cooking spray.
3. Place the potatoes in the baking dish and toss them with the shitake mushrooms. Top the mixture with Brie cubes.
4. In a medium bowl, whisk the cream with the garlic, thyme, salt, and pepper. Pour the mixture over the potatoes.
5. Cover and bake for 30 minutes. Remove the cover, and top the potatoes with the Parmesan cheese and bread crumbs.
6. Bake uncovered for an additional 15 minutes or until light brown and bubbly. Switch the oven rack to the top rung and set the oven temperature to broil. Brown the top of the potatoes. Serve immediately.

ROASTED POTATOES WITH MINTED GARLIC

When mint, one of summer's most popular herbs, is abundant in the garden, this recipe is often a complementary accompaniment to grilled meats, summer salads, and side dishes. The warm potatoes sop up a few of my favorite basic and flavorful pantry items—olive oil, garlic, salt, and pepper. Then freshly picked mint is added for a burst of flavor.

6 servings

8 medium russet potatoes
¼ cup olive oil
4 cloves garlic, minced
1 teaspoon salt
A few grindings of black pepper
2 tablespoons fresh mint, chopped

1. Preheat the oven to 375°F.
2. Cook the whole potatoes for 1 hour or until tender when pierced with a fork.
3. While the potatoes are cooking, prepare the garlic and mint mixture. In a small bowl, whisk the olive oil, minced garlic, salt, and pepper. Add the mint and combine until well blended.
4. When the potatoes are cool enough to handle, quarter them or cut into desired-size pieces. Transfer the potatoes to a large bowl.
5. Drizzle the garlic and mint mixture over the warm potatoes, and gently toss. Serve immediately or cover tightly and keep the potatoes at room temperature until serving time.

SIMPLE CREAMY POTATOES

Comfort food extraordinaire! This crowd-pleasing side dish complements pork, chicken, lamb, beef, and a variety of vegetables. The best potatoes to use in this recipe are waxy or all-purpose potatoes. They hold their shape when boiled and have a nice creamy texture once cooked. Waxy and all-purpose potatoes are typically thin skinned and are reddish, golden, or purple.

4 servings

4 medium potatoes, unpeeled and cut into bite-sized cubes
1 tablespoon neutral oil (expeller-pressed canola, high-oleic safflower, or sunflower oil)
4 garlic cloves, crushed
½ cup mascarpone cheese
¼ cup heavy cream
½ teaspoon salt
A few grindings of black pepper

1. Cook the potatoes in a large pot of boiling salted water for 5 to 10 minutes or until fork-tender. Drain them, return them to the pot, cover, and keep warm.
2. In a large skillet, heat the oil over medium-low heat. Add the crushed garlic and cook for about 1 minute or until fragrant. Add the mascarpone cheese and cream, and whisk until smooth and well combined. Add the salt, pepper, and cooked potatoes to the cream mixture. Stir until well combined and heated through. Serve immediately.

ROASTED CURRIED POTATOES

This recipe is similar to roasted potatoes with minted garlic on page 103. Here, a generous amount of curry is the hero for flavoring the potatoes. The key to optimum flavor is to toss the hot potatoes with the remaining ingredients. The heat helps to release all the spices' flavors.

6 servings

8 medium russet potatoes
¼ cup olive oil
1 tablespoon dried minced onion
3 teaspoons curry powder
1 teaspoon salt
Several grindings of black pepper

1. Preheat the oven to 375°F.
2. Bake the whole potatoes for 1 hour or until tender when pierced with a fork.
3. While the potatoes are cooking, prepare the curry mixture. In a small bowl, whisk the olive oil, minced onion, curry powder, salt, and pepper until well blended.
4. While the potatoes are still hot, quarter them or cut them into desired-size pieces. To keep from burning your hand, partially cover the potato with a pot holder. Transfer the potatoes to a large bowl.
5. Pour the curry mixture over the warm potatoes and gently toss to combine. Serve immediately or cover and keep the potatoes at room temperature until serving time.

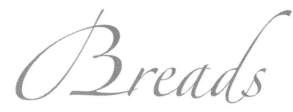

Breads

RUSTIC BREADS
GRAIN AND SEED BREADS
PIZZA CRUST

For me, one of the greatest culinary rewards is that of bread-making. It captures my senses in every way, and I have yet to find anyone who can resist the aroma of baking bread as it wafts from the kitchen. In this chapter, you will find an unusual and eclectic group of recipes. There are two recipes for pizza crust—thin crust that comes together in a little under an hour and thick crust with a dough that needs to be refrigerated overnight. Many of the recipes in this chapter incorporate interesting grains, seeds, and flours—for example, tricolor quinoa, whole-grain pilaf, oatmeal, chia, hemp, flaxseeds, spelt, rye, and wheat germ. My favorites? A divine recipe for cranberry autumn spice bread, grain and seed bread, a surprising loaf that includes spaghetti squash, and my cast-iron honey-glazed cornbread.

If you haven't tried bread-making, I encourage you to try some of these recipes. Keep in mind that making bread is not an exact science; there is no right or wrong. It is more of an art form in which each loaf is a one-of-a-kind masterpiece. To help get you started, I've included some tips for successful bread-making.

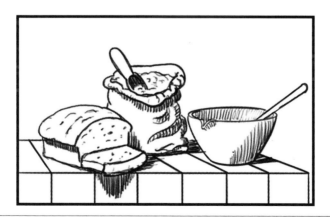

RECIPE INDEX

RUSTIC BREADS

No-Knead, All-Purpose, Country-Style Bread 110

Cranberry Autumn Spice Bread 111-112

Molasses-Tinged Pumpernickel Raisin Bread 113-114

Cast-Iron Honey-Glazed Corn Bread 115

Basic White Bread 116

All-Purpose Bread 117-118

Buttermilk Bread 119

Pumpkin Yeast Bread 120-121

Spaghetti Squash Bread 122

GRAIN AND SEED BREADS

Dual Seed Tricolor Quinoa Bread 123-124

Spelt Bread with Hemp Seeds 125

Seven Whole Grain Bread 126-127

Chia Quinoa Bread 128-129

Oatmeal Bread 130

Grain and Seed Bread 131-132

PIZZA CRUST

Thick Crust Pizza 133-134

Thin Crust Pizza 135

SUCCESSFUL BREAD-MAKING TIPS

- It's best if all ingredients are at room temperature.

- The yeast should be fresh—check the expiration date before using. Yeast generally will not proof if the temperature of the liquid added is too cold or too hot. I use the inside of my wrist (an area that's sensitive to hot and cold) for testing the temperature of the liquid. It should be no hotter than what you would give a baby. Yeast requires a warm, damp environment to proof, as well as the addition of food (honey or sugar). Proofing yeast is like watching a chemistry experiment—ingredients reacting to other ingredients. The process takes 5 to 10 minutes, and the result should be a foamy and/or bubbly mixture.

- Dough can be quite temperamental, and typically performs according to the weather conditions in your kitchen. Humidity makes for stickier dough, which means you'll need to add more flour while kneading. Colder/dryer conditions will require less flour during this process. When adding flour during the kneading process, measurements are not exact. Add flour until your dough is smooth and elastic. You will find many techniques for kneading dough; the perfect technique is the one that works best for you.

- Most bread dough requires at least two risings. During this process, dough should be in a warm environment, free of cold drafts. Suitable places include the top of a warm radiator, near something warming on the stove or, on a warm day, in natural sunlight. Rising times vary; on average, expect about 1 hour per rising.

- After a rising, you will always be asked to "punch down" the dough. Punching down is not so much about the act of punching as it is about the act of flattening. Use your fist or outstretched hand to push down the dough to deflate it.

NO-KNEAD, ALL-PURPOSE, COUNTRY-STYLE BREAD

This finely textured loaf has only one rising, just 45 minutes—more of a settling and partial rising than a double-in-size rising—all the sooner to delve into slices of warm bread slathered with butter.

1 loaf

5 cups unbleached all-purpose flour
2 packages active dry yeast
1 tablespoon granulated sugar
1 tablespoon salt
½ teaspoon baking soda
2 cups warm milk
½ cup warm water

1. Generously oil a 9 x 5 x 3-inch loaf pan with cooking spray. Dust the pan with cornmeal. Set aside.
2. In the large bowl of a stand mixer, combine 2 cups of all-purpose flour with the yeast, sugar, salt, and baking soda. Add the warm milk and water and beat on low speed for about 30 seconds. Increase the speed to high and beat for about 3 minutes. Stir in the remaining flour—the batter will be stiff and sticky.
3. Transfer the dough to the prepared pan. Cover the pan with a kitchen towel and let the dough rest for about 45 minutes.
4. Preheat the oven to 375°F.
5. Bake the loaf for 35 to 45 minutes or until golden brown or until the bread sounds hollow when tapped on the top and bottom. To crisp the crust, remove the loaf from the bread pan and place the loaf on the oven rack, and bake for 1 to 2 minutes. Place the loaf on a wire rack and allow it to cool before slicing.

CRANBERRY AUTUMN SPICE BREAD

This autumn-inspired loaf makes fantastic turkey sandwiches, and slices are delicious toasted and flooded with butter. Plan accordingly; this recipe uses the autumn spice blend (see page 148). If you're not inclined to make the blend, Spice Hunter Hot Buttered Rum Mix, available online, is a fine replacement.

1 loaf

1½ cups dried cranberries
2 cups water
1 package active dry yeast
½ cup warm water
¼ cup neutral oil (expeller-pressed canola, high-oleic safflower, or sunflower oil)
1½ teaspoons salt
½ cup whole wheat flour
3 to 3½ cups all-purpose flour
¼ cup autumn spice blend

1. In a medium saucepan, combine the cranberries with the water. Bring the mixture to a boil, reduce the heat to simmer, and simmer for 5 minutes. Drain the cranberries and reserve the cranberry water. Set aside.
2. In a large bowl, combine the warm water with the yeast and stir until the yeast dissolves. Allow the yeast to proof. Add the reserved cranberry water, oil, salt, whole wheat flour, and 1 cup of all-purpose flour to the mixture, and stir until well combined. Add the cranberries and stir until well distributed. Add the remaining all-purpose flour, 1 cup at a time. When the dough begins to pull away from the sides of the bowl, transfer it to a floured surface. Knead the dough, adding more flour to keep it from sticking to the work surface, until the dough is smooth and elastic.
3. Coat a large bowl with cooking spray. Transfer the dough to the prepared bowl and turn to coat all surfaces. Cover with a kitchen towel and let it rise in a warm, draft-free place until double in bulk, about 1 hour.
4. Punch the dough down. Transfer to a floured board and let the dough rest for about 5 minutes.
5. Coat a 9 x 5 x 3-inch pan with cooking spray.

6. Roll the dough into a rectangle about 7 x 15 inches. Sprinkle the dough with the autumn spice blend. Using the palm of your hand, press the mixture into the dough. Roll the dough up tightly, and tuck each end under. Carefully transfer the loaf, seam side down, to the prepared pan. Cover with a kitchen towel and let it rise until the dough comes up over the top of the pan, about 1½ to 2 hours.
7. Preheat the oven to 400°F.
8. Bake the bread for 10 minutes, then reduce the oven temperature to 350°F and continue to bake for another 20 minutes or until the bread sounds hollow when tapped on the top and bottom. Remove the bread from the pan, return the loaf to the oven, and bake for 1 to 2 minutes to brown the crust. Transfer the bread to a wire rack to cool before slicing.

MOLASSES-TINGED PUMPERNICKEL RAISIN BREAD

This is a hearty loaf of bread that's got great texture. It's a versatile bread that can be turned into French toast or enjoyed with a variety of cheeses, soups, or stews, and it makes a memorable bread for sandwiches. Plan accordingly; this dough has three risings, all more than the typical 1-hour rising time.

2 loaves

1½ cups warm water
½ cup molasses
1 package active dry yeast
1 tablespoon salt
⅛ cup cocoa powder
2 cups rye flour
2 cups whole wheat flour
½ cup unbleached all-purpose flour
1 cup raisins, roughly chopped

1. In a large bowl, combine the warm water with the molasses. Add the yeast and stir to dissolve. Let the mixture stand for about 10 minutes, or until slightly foamy. Add the salt, cocoa, and rye flour to the molasses/yeast mixture. Stir until well combined. Add the whole wheat flour ½ cup at a time, stirring well after each addition. Add the all-purpose flour. When the dough begins to pull away from the sides of the bowl, transfer to a floured surface and knead (using more flour if necessary) for about 10 minutes or until smooth and elastic.
2. Coat a large bowl with cooking spray. Add the dough and turn to coat all the surfaces. Cover with a kitchen towel and let the dough rise in a warm, draft-free place until it is tripled in bulk, about 3 hours.
3. Punch the dough down and turn out onto a lightly floured surface. Flatten the dough into a rectangle and sprinkle with raisins. Gather the dough and knead it for about 5 minutes, making certain to distribute the raisins.
4. Return the dough to the oiled bowl and cover with a kitchen towel. Let the dough rise until double in bulk, about 1½ hours.

5. Coat two 9 x 5 x 3-inch loaf pans with cooking spray.

6. Punch the dough down, cut the dough in half, and form into 2 rounds. Place each round in the prepared pans. Cover the pans with a kitchen towel and let the dough rise until double in bulk, about 1 hour.

7. Preheat the oven to 400°F.

8. Bake the bread for 30 minutes or until the loaves are dark brown and sound hollow when tapped on the top and bottom. Transfer the bread to a wire rack to cool before slicing.

CAST-IRON HONEY-GLAZED CORN BREAD

I rely on this moist and delicious corn bread recipe when I need a quick bread. The butter and honey act like a glaze, like thin icing on a cake. If you don't have a cast-iron skillet, you can use an 11 x 7 x 2-inch baking dish. Whenever I have any leftover corn bread, I cut it in half crosswise, butter the cut side, and cook the buttered side in a skillet until toasty brown in spots. Then for a memorable breakfast, I top the corn bread with a poached egg. Huzzah!

8 servings

1¼ cups unbleached all-purpose flour
¾ cup yellow-corn flour
3 tablespoons granulated sugar
5 teaspoons baking powder
¾ teaspoon salt
1 egg
1¼ cups buttermilk
2 tablespoons neutral oil (expeller-pressed canola, high-oleic safflower, or
*   sunflower oil)*
1 tablespoon butter
Honey

1. Preheat the oven to 350°F.
2. Generously coat a 10-inch cast-iron skillet with cooking spray.
3. Combine the flour, corn flour, sugar, baking powder, and salt in a large bowl.
4. In a medium bowl, whisk the egg with the buttermilk and oil. Make a well in the center of the dry ingredients and add the liquid mixture. Stir just to combine.
5. Transfer the batter to the prepared skillet, and bake for 25 to 30 minutes (check after 25 minutes), or until a toothpick inserted in the center comes out clean.
6. Switch the oven temperature to broil and brown the top for 1 to 2 minutes. While the corn bread is hot, spread the butter evenly over the top, drizzle with a generous amount of the honey, and spread it evenly across the top. Serve immediately.

BASIC WHITE BREAD

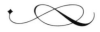

This is an all-purpose, go-to loaf that makes a fine sandwich bread and is lovely to serve with soup.

2 loaves

1 package active dry yeast
1 teaspoon granulated sugar
1⅔ cups warm water
1½ teaspoons salt
3½ cups unbleached all-purpose flour

1. In a large bowl, combine the yeast, sugar, and ⅓ cup of warm water. Stir until the yeast dissolves. Proof the yeast for 5 to 15 minutes.
2. After the yeast has proofed, add salt and the remaining 1⅓ cups warm water to the bowl. Add the flour ½ cup at a time, stirring well after each addition. When the dough begins to pull away from the sides of the bowl, turn out onto a lightly floured surface. Add flour as needed to keep the dough from sticking to the work surface and knead until the bread is smooth and elastic.
3. Coat a large bowl with cooking spray. Transfer the dough to the bowl and coat all the surfaces with oil. Cover with a kitchen towel and allow the dough to rise for about 1 hour.
4. Coat two 9 x 5 x 3-inch bread pans with cooking spray.
5. Punch the dough down, cut in half, and shape into 2 rounds. Place the loaves in the prepared pans. Cover the loaves with a kitchen towel and let them rise for about 1 hour.
6. Preheat the oven to 450°F.
7. Bake the bread for 10 minutes. Reduce the oven temperature to 350°F and bake an additional 20 minutes or until the bread sounds hollow when tapped on the top and bottom. To crisp the crust, remove the loaves from the bread pans, place them on the oven rack, and bake for 1 to 2 minutes. Place the loaves on a wire rack and allow them to cool before slicing.

ALL-PURPOSE BREAD

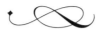

This is a delicious loaf that is wonderful for just about any kind of sandwich. It's also marvelous toasted and spread with butter and jam.

2 loaves

2 packages active dry yeast
½ cup warm water
1 tablespoon granulated sugar
1 cup water
1 teaspoon salt
½ cup corn flour
2 teaspoons salt
2 cups warm water
2 tablespoons honey
½ cup spelt flour
½ cup whole wheat flour
4 to 5 cups unbleached all-purpose flour

1. Combine the yeast with the warm water and sugar in a large bowl. Allow the mixture to proof for about 5 minutes.
2. In a medium saucepan, bring 1 cup of water to a boil. Add 1 teaspoon salt and gradually add the corn flour. (Be cautious; sometimes the hot mixture splatters.) Lower the heat to a simmer and cook for about 1 minute, stirring vigorously. Cool the mixture for about 5 minutes, then transfer to the bowl with the yeast mixture. Stir until well combined.
3. Add the salt, water, honey, spelt flour, and whole wheat flour. Stir until the ingredients are incorporated. Add the all-purpose flour, 1 cup at a time, stirring well after each addition. When the mixture begins to pull away from the sides of the bowl, transfer the dough to a floured surface and knead for about 10 minutes or until smooth and elastic.
4. Coat a large bowl with cooking spray. Add the dough and turn to coat all surfaces. Cover with a kitchen towel and let the dough rise in a warm, draft-free place until double in bulk, about 1 hour.
5. Coat two 9 x 5 x 3-inch loaf pans with cooking spray.
6. Punch the dough down, cut the dough in half, and shape into 2 rounds. Place the loaves in the prepared pans. Cover the pans with a kitchen towel and let the dough rise until double in bulk, about 1 hour.

7. Preheat the oven to 425°F.

8. Bake the bread for 10 minutes. Reduce the oven temperature to 350°F and bake an additional 20 to 25 minutes or until the loaves are light brown and sound hollow when tapped on the top and bottom. Transfer the loaves to a wire rack and allow the bread to cool before slicing.

BUTTERMILK BREAD

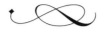

This loaf makes great sandwich bread.

2 loaves

2 packages active dry yeast
1 tablespoon granulated sugar
½ cup warm water
3½ cups unbleached all-purpose flour
½ cup spelt flour
1 tablespoon salt
3 tablespoons neutral oil (expeller-pressed canola, high-oleic safflower, or
sunflower oil)
1½ cups buttermilk

1. Combine the yeast, sugar, and warm water in a medium bowl. Stir until the yeast dissolves. Proof the yeast for about 5 minutes.
2. In a large bowl, combine the all-purpose flour with the spelt flour and salt. Add the oil and buttermilk and mix until incorporated. Add the yeast mixture and stir until combined.
3. Turn out onto a lightly floured surface and knead for about 10 minutes or until smooth and elastic. Add more all-purpose flour as needed to keep the dough from sticking to the work surface.
4. Coat a large bowl with cooking spray. Add the dough and turn to coat all surfaces. Cover the dough with a kitchen towel and let it rise in a warm, draft-free place until double in bulk, about 1 hour.
5. Coat two 9 x 5 x 3-inch loaf pans with cooking spray.
6. Punch the dough down, transfer to a floured surface, and knead for 1 to 2 minutes. Cut the dough in half, form each half into a round, and place in the prepared loaf pans. Cover the loaves with a kitchen towel and let the dough rise until double in bulk, about 1 hour.
7. Preheat the oven to 350°F.
8. Bake the bread for 40 minutes or until the loaves are light brown and sound hollow when tapped on the top and bottom. Allow the loaves to cool on a wire rack before slicing.

PUMPKIN YEAST BREAD

This recipe is the result of some leftover pumpkin—specifically, canned pure pumpkin. It's a lovely loaf with a beautiful pale burnt-orange color. The flavor is like pumpkin itself—mellow. Slather warm or toasted slices with butter. You can also use it for sandwiches or serve with steaming bowls of soup. It also makes delicious Thanksgiving stuffing. When I use this bread for our holiday stuffing, I use one part pumpkin yeast bread, one part corn bread, and one part of either the basic, all-purpose, or buttermilk bread recipes (see Index for page references).

2 loaves

2 packages active dry yeast
1 teaspoon granulated sugar
½ cup warm water
1¼ cups cooked pure pumpkin, mashed
1 cup buttermilk
2 tablespoons neutral oil (expeller-pressed canola, high-oleic safflower, or
  sunflower oil)
¼ cup brown sugar
3 teaspoons salt
½ cup wheat germ
2 cups whole wheat flour
3 cups unbleached all-purpose flour

1. Combine the yeast, sugar, and warm water in a large bowl. Stir the mixture until the yeast dissolves. Proof the yeast for 5 to 15 minutes.
2. Add the pumpkin, buttermilk, oil, brown sugar, salt, and wheat germ to the yeast mixture. Add the whole wheat flour 1 cup at a time, stirring well after each addition. Add the all-purpose flour, 1 cup at a time. After you've added the second cup of all-purpose flour and the dough begins to pull away from the sides of the bowl, turn out to a floured board and knead the dough for about 10 minutes, adding more flour as necessary to keep it from sticking to the surface. Knead until the dough is smooth and elastic, about 10 minutes.
3. Coat a large bowl with cooking spray. Transfer the dough to the prepared bowl and coat all surfaces with the oil. Cover the bowl with a kitchen towel and allow the dough to rise for about 1 hour.
4. Punch the dough down and divide it in half.

5. Coat two 9 x 5 x 3-inch bread pans with cooking spray.

6. Form each half into a round and place in the prepared pans. Cover the loaves with a kitchen towel and let them rise until doubled in bulk, about 30 minutes.

7. Preheat the oven to 375°F.

8. Bake the bread for 25 to 30 minutes or until golden brown. Remove the bread from the pans and allow the loaves to cool on a wire rack for about 10 minutes before slicing.

Spaghetti Squash Bread

This recipe is the result of some leftover spaghetti squash. It's a lovely loaf with a beautiful buttery color. The flavor is like spaghetti squash itself—mellow. Slather warm slices with butter or toast it. You can also use it for sandwiches or serve with steaming bowls of soup. If you don't have any leftover spaghetti squash and want to make this bread, spaghetti squash is super-simple to cook. Instructions for cooking can be found in the Product Reference Guide, page 233.

1 loaf

1 package active dry yeast
1 tablespoon honey
1¼ cups warm water
1 cup cooked spaghetti squash, finely chopped
1½ teaspoons salt
½ cup wheat germ
½ cup whole wheat flour
3 cups unbleached all-purpose flour

1. In a large bowl, combine the yeast, honey, and ¼ cup of the warm water. Stir the mixture until the yeast dissolves. Proof the yeast for 5 to 15 minutes.
2. Add the remaining water, squash, salt, wheat germ, and whole wheat flour to the yeast mixture. Add the all-purpose flour, 1 cup at a time. When the dough begins to pull away from the sides of the bowl, turn out onto a floured board and knead the dough for about 10 minutes, adding more all-purpose flour to keep the dough from sticking to the surface. Knead for about 10 minutes, or until the dough is smooth and elastic.
3. Coat a large bowl with cooking spray. Transfer the dough to the prepared bowl and coat all surfaces with the oil. Cover the bowl with a kitchen towel and allow the dough to rise for about 1 hour.
4. Punch the dough down and let it rest while you prepare the bread pan.
5. Coat a 9 x 5 x 3-inch bread pan with cooking spray.
6. Form the dough into a round and place in the prepared pan. Cover the loaf with a kitchen towel and let it rise for about 30 minutes, or until doubled in bulk.
7. Preheat the oven to 375°F.
8. Bake for 25 to 30 minutes or until golden brown. Remove the bread from the pan and allow it to cool on a wire rack for about 10 minutes before slicing.

DUAL SEED
TRICOLOR QUINOA BREAD

This is a great bread to use for sandwiches, a good accompaniment to a variety of soups, and delicious toasted.

1 loaf

½ cup water
⅓ cup tricolor quinoa
1 package active dry yeast
1 teaspoon granulated sugar
½ cup warm water
1 teaspoon salt
1 cup buttermilk
½ cup hemp seeds
¼ cup ground flaxseeds
3½ to 4 cups unbleached all-purpose flour

1. Bring the water to boil in a small pan. Stir in the quinoa, remove from heat, cover, and set aside.
2. Combine the yeast with the sugar in a large bowl. Add the water and stir until the yeast dissolves. Proof the yeast for about 5 minutes. Add the salt, buttermilk, hemp seeds, cooked quinoa, and ground flaxseeds to the yeast mixture. Stir until well combined. Add the all-purpose flour, 1 cup at a time, stirring well after each addition. When the dough begins to pull away from the sides of the bowl, turn out onto a lightly floured surface. Knead the dough for about 10 minutes or until smooth and elastic. Add the all-purpose flour as needed to keep the dough from sticking to the work surface.
3. Coat a large bowl with cooking spray. Add the dough and turn to coat all the surfaces. Cover with a kitchen towel and let the dough rise in a warm, draft-free place for about 1 hour or until double in bulk.
4. Coat a 9 x 5 x 3-inch loaf pan with cooking spray.
5. Punch the dough down, transfer to a floured surface, and knead for 1 to 2 minutes. Form the dough into a round and place in the prepared pan. Cover the loaf pan with a kitchen towel and let the dough rise for about 1 hour, or until double in bulk.
6. Preheat the oven to 425°F.

7. Bake the bread in the center of the oven for 10 minutes. Reduce the oven temperature to 350°F and cook an additional 20 minutes. Remove the bread from the pan, return it to the oven, and bake for 1 to 2 minutes to crisp the bottom and sides. Allow the bread to cool on a wire rack before slicing.

SPELT BREAD WITH HEMP SEEDS

Hemp seeds give this bread a delightfully subtle crunch.

2 loaves

1 package active dry yeast
1 teaspoon granulated sugar
1⅔ cups warm water
1½ teaspoons salt
½ cup hemp seeds
½ cup spelt flour
½ cup rye flour
2½ cups unbleached all-purpose flour

1. In a large bowl, combine the yeast, sugar, and ⅓ cup of warm water. Stir until the yeast dissolves. Proof the yeast for 5 to 10 minutes. Add the salt and remaining warm water to the bowl. Add the hemp seeds, spelt flour, and rye flour, and stir until well combined. Add the all-purpose flour, ½ cup at a time, stirring well after each addition. When the dough begins to pull away from the sides of the bowl, turn out onto a lightly floured surface. Knead until the dough is smooth and elastic. Add the all-purpose flour as needed to keep the dough from sticking to the work surface.
2. Coat a large bowl with cooking spray. Transfer the dough to the bowl and coat all surfaces with oil. Cover with a kitchen towel and allow the dough to rise for about 1 hour.
3. Punch the dough down and let it rest while you prepare the bread pans.
4. Coat two 9 x 5 x 3-inch bread pans with cooking spray. Cut the dough in half and form each piece into a round. Place the dough in the prepared pans. Cover the loaves with a kitchen towel and let them rise for about 1 hour.
5. Preheat the oven to 450°F.
6. Bake the bread for 10 minutes. Reduce the oven temperature to 350°F and bake for an additional 20 minutes or until the bread sounds hollow when tapped on the top and the bottom. Remove the loaves from the bread pans and place them on the oven rack. Bake for 1 to 2 minutes to crisp the bottom and sides of the bread. Place the loaves on a wire rack to cool before slicing.

SEVEN WHOLE GRAIN BREAD

The seven whole grain pilaf (Kashi brand) is a delicious and nutrient-rich mixture of whole oats, brown rice, rye, hard red wheat, triticale, buckwheat, barley, and sesame seeds. The addition of the cooked pilaf turns out a nicely textured, flavorful, and interesting bread.

2 loaves

2 cups water
1 cup whole grain pilaf
1 package active dry yeast
1 teaspoon honey
1¼ cups warm water
¼ cup honey
1 cup buttermilk
1 tablespoon salt
1 cup whole wheat flour
3 to 3½ cups unbleached all-purpose flour

1. In a medium pan, bring the water to a boil. Add the whole grain pilaf, cover, reduce the heat to medium, and cook for about 25 minutes or until the water is absorbed. Set aside.

2. Combine the yeast, honey, and ¼ cup of the warm water in a large bowl. Stir until the yeast dissolves. Proof the mixture for about 5 minutes.

3. Add the remaining water, honey, buttermilk, salt, and cooked whole grain pilaf. Stir until well combined.

4. Add the whole wheat flour and mix well. Add 2 cups of all-purpose flour and mix well. Continue to stir, adding a little flour at a time. When the dough begins to pull away from the sides of the bowl, turn out onto a floured surface and knead for 5 to 7 minutes or until the dough becomes smooth and elastic.

5. Coat a large bowl with cooking spray. Add the dough and turn to coat all the surfaces. Cover with a kitchen towel and let the dough rise in a warm, draft-free place for 1 to 1½ hours or until double in bulk.

6. Coat two 9 x 5 x 3-inch loaf pans with cooking spray.

7. Punch the dough down and cut in half. Shape each half into two rounds. If the dough is sticky, dust it with flour. Place the dough in the prepared loaf pans. Cover the pans with a kitchen towel and let the dough rise for about 1 hour or until double in bulk.

8. Preheat the oven to 425°F.

9. Bake the bread for 10 minutes. Reduce the oven temperature to 350°F and bake an additional 20 to 25 minutes or until the loaves are light brown and sound hollow when tapped on the top and bottom. Remove the bread from the pans and place on the oven rack. Bake for an additional 2 to 3 minutes to crisp the crust. Transfer to a wire rack and allow the bread to cool before slicing.

CHIA QUINOA BREAD

This is a great bread for sandwiches. It's a good accompaniment to a variety of soups and is delicious toasted. The nutrient-rich chia seeds give this bread a welcome crunch.

1 loaf

½ cup water
⅓ cup plain quinoa
1 package active dry yeast
1 teaspoon granulated sugar
½ cup warm water
1 teaspoon salt
1 cup buttermilk
3 tablespoons chia seeds
½ cup spelt flour
2½ cups unbleached all-purpose flour

1. Bring the water to boil in a small pan. Stir in the quinoa, remove from heat, cover, and set aside.

2. Combine the yeast, sugar, and water in a large bowl. Stir until the yeast dissolves. Proof the yeast for about 5 minutes. Add the salt, buttermilk, chia seeds, and cooked quinoa to the yeast mixture. Stir until well combined. Add the spelt flour and 1 cup all-purpose flour, and stir until incorporated. Add another cup of all-purpose flour and stir to combine. When the dough begins to pull away from the sides of the bowl, turn out onto a lightly floured surface. Knead the dough for about 10 minutes or until smooth and elastic. Add more all-purpose flour as needed to keep the dough from sticking to the work surface.

3. Coat a large bowl with cooking spray. Add the dough and turn to coat all the surfaces. Cover with a kitchen towel and let the dough rise in a warm, draft-free place for 1 hour or until double in bulk.

4. Coat a 9 x 5 x 3-inch loaf pan with cooking spray.

5. Punch the dough down, transfer to a floured surface, and knead for 1 to 2 minutes. Shape the dough into a round, folding in the ends and then folding in the sides. Place in the prepared loaf pan. Cover the pan with a kitchen towel and let the dough rise for 1 hour or until double in bulk.

6. Preheat the oven to 425°F.

7. Bake the bread in the center of the oven for 10 minutes. Reduce the oven temperature to 350°F and bake for an additional 20 minutes. Remove the bread from the pan, return it to the oven, and bake for 1 to 2 minutes to crisp the bottom and sides. Allow the bread to cool on a wire rack before slicing.

OATMEAL BREAD

This pleasant loaf is lovely to serve with steaming bowls of hearty soup and is great for sandwiches. It's excellent toasted and slathered with butter. Take note: The oats are soaked in the water for 2 hours before being added to the yeast mixture.

2 loaves

2 cups quick-cooking oats
2 cups water
1 package active dry yeast
¾ cup warm water
1 teaspoon granulated sugar
¼ cup neutral oil (expeller-pressed canola, high-oleic safflower, or sunflower oil)
1 teaspoon salt
4 cups unbleached all-purpose flour

1. Combine the quick-cooking oats and water in a large bowl. Cover and let stand at room temperature for about 2 hours.
2. In a small bowl, dissolve the yeast in the water, and add the sugar. Allow the mixture to proof for about 5 minutes.
3. Add the yeast mixture to the soaked oatmeal mixture. Add the oil and salt, and stir until well combined. Add the flour, 1 cup at a time. When the dough begins to pull away from the sides of the bowl, transfer it to a floured surface. Knead the dough for 7 to 10 minutes or until it's smooth and elastic. Add flour, as needed, to keep the dough from sticking to the work surface.
4. Coat a large bowl with cooking spray. Place the dough in the bowl and turn it to coat all the surfaces. Cover with a kitchen towel and let it rise in a warm, draft-free place for 1 hour or until double in bulk.
5. Coat two 9 x 5 x 3-inch loaf pans with cooking spray.
6. Punch the dough down and transfer to a lightly floured work surface. Cut the dough in half and shape into 2 rounds. Place each round in the prepared pans. Cover the pans with a kitchen towel and let the dough rise for about an hour.
7. Preheat the oven to 425°F.
8. Bake the bread for 10 minutes, reduce the oven temperature to 350°F, and bake an additional 20 minutes or until the loaves sound hollow when tapped on the top and bottom. Transfer the bread to a wire rack and allow the bread to cool before slicing.

GRAIN AND SEED BREAD

This is a multi-purpose bread that is great to use for sandwiches. It's also delicious toasted. The oatmeal gives this loaf a marvelous texture, and the cooked quinoa makes it spongy, almost like very fresh white bread.

1 loaf

½ cup water
⅓ cup plain quinoa
1 package active dry yeast
1 teaspoon granulated sugar
½ cup warm water
2 teaspoons salt
1 cup buttermilk
½ cup raw quick-cooking oatmeal
1 cup quinoa, cooked
¼ cup ground flaxseed
2 to 3 cups unbleached all-purpose flour

1. Bring the water to a boil in a small pan. Stir in the quinoa, remove from heat, cover, and set aside for 5 minutes.
2. In a large bowl, combine the yeast, sugar, and water. Stir until the yeast dissolves. Proof the yeast for about 5 minutes. Add the salt, buttermilk, oatmeal, cooked quinoa, and flaxseed to the yeast mixture. Stir until well combined. Add flour, 1 cup at a time, stirring well after each addition. When the dough begins to pull away from the sides of the bowl, turn out onto a lightly floured surface. Knead for about 10 minutes or until smooth and elastic. Add more flour, as needed, to keep the dough from sticking to the work surface.
3. Coat a large bowl with cooking spray. Add the dough and turn to coat all the surfaces. Cover the dough with a kitchen towel and let it rise in a warm, draft-free place for 1 hour or until double in bulk.
4. Coat a 9 x 5 x 3-inch loaf pan with cooking spray.
5. Punch the dough down, transfer to a floured surface, and knead for about 1 to 2 minutes. Form the dough into a round, folding in the ends and then folding in the sides. Place in the prepared loaf pan. Cover the pan with a kitchen towel and let the dough rise for 1 hour or until double in bulk.
6. Preheat the oven to 425°F.

7. Bake the bread for 10 minutes. Reduce the oven temperature to 350°F and bake for an additional 20 minutes. Remove the bread from the pan, return it to the oven, and bake for 1 to 2 minutes to crisp the sides and bottom. Allow the bread to cool on a wire rack before slicing.

THICK CRUST PIZZA

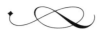

I'm typically not one to fool around with delicious food that talented restaurant chefs have created and perfected—like the makers at Matthew's Pizza in Baltimore. After so many years of eating their pizza, coupled with the culinary knowledge I've learned during my decades-long food career and the food science it sometimes requires, I was challenged to give it a try. I started by making a focaccia-like dough because it's got a somewhat airy texture like Matthew's. I decided to initially cook the pizzas in my well-seasoned cast-iron skillets on the stovetop, and then finish baking them in the oven. We were pleased with the results. Take note: The dough gets refrigerated overnight.

2 (10-inch) pizzas

2¾ cups unbleached all-purpose flour
1 tablespoon granulated sugar
1 package active dry yeast
1 teaspoon salt
1¼ cups cold water
3 tablespoons olive oil, plus more for drizzling over the finished pizzas
½ to 1 cup pizza sauce
⅔ cup Parmesan Reggiano cheese, freshly grated
A few grindings of black pepper

1. Combine the flour, sugar, yeast, salt, and water in a large bowl. Mix the ingredients with your hands. Knead the dough for about 3 minutes. Note: The dough will be extremely sticky. Let the dough rest for about 5 minutes. Knead for another 2 to 3 minutes. The dough will be somewhat smooth, but still very sticky. Add 1 tablespoon olive oil and turn the dough to coat all the surfaces. Grab a large portion of the dough with one hand, hold it above the bowl, and allow it to stretch out until it doubles in size. Repeat this process three more times. Cover the bowl with plastic wrap, cover with a kitchen towel, and refrigerate the dough overnight.
2. Remove the dough from the refrigerator and, using a rubber spatula, transfer it to a rimmed baking sheet that has been brushed with olive oil. Let the dough rest at room temperature for about 20 minutes.
3. Place 1 tablespoon of olive oil into each cast-iron skillet and brush the bottom of the skillet with the oil. Cut the dough in half and place in each skillet. Starting in the center of the dough, splay your fingers and make indentations over the surface of the dough, creating hollows as the dough is moved down and out toward the edges of the skillet.

If the dough resists, let it rest for 5 minutes. (Don't worry if it doesn't reach the edge of the skillet.) Place a kitchen towel over the dough and let it rest for 1 hour.

4. After the dough has rested, preheat the oven to 500°F.

5. Spread ½ cup of the pizza sauce (or less depending on your sauce preference) over the top of each piece of dough. You don't need to leave a border because as the pizza rises from the heat on the stovetop and in the oven, the edges swell, moving the sauce more toward the center. Sprinkle ⅓ cup of Parmesan cheese over the sauce on each pizza.

6. If using an electric stove, the heating element of the burner should be the same size as the skillet. Set the stovetop burner dial to medium heat; if your dials are numbered, set the dial to 4. Place the skillet on the burner. Cook the pizza for 5 to 7 minutes or until golden on the bottom. Stovetop times vary—once cast iron is hot, it holds its heat. To make sure you don't burn the bottom of the crust, frequently check using a metal spatula to lift the crust. Transfer the skillets to the oven and bake for 5 to 8 minutes or until the crust is light brown and the pizza is bubbly.

7. Carefully transfer the pizza to a platter, drizzle with olive oil, and lightly season with pepper. Cut into wedges and serve immediately.

THIN CRUST PIZZA

This recipe came to me from a friend who had been trying to master thin crust pizza dough—she refuses to buy commercially made pizza for her son, who loves pizza. It's a simple recipe and an easy dough to work with. The amounts of tomato sauce, cheese, and additional toppings are based on your preferences.

2 (10-to-12-inch) pizzas

1 package active dry yeast
1 teaspoon honey
⅔ cup warm water
½ teaspoon salt
About 1¼ cups unbleached all-purpose flour
Pizza sauce
Freshly shredded mozzarella cheese
Additional toppings, if desired

1. In a large bowl, combine the yeast with the honey and ⅓ cup of the water. Allow the yeast to proof for about 5 minutes. Add the remaining ⅓ cup of water, salt, and 1 cup of flour. Stir to combine the ingredients.
2. Transfer the dough to a floured surface and knead until the dough is smooth and elastic. Add more flour as needed to keep the dough from sticking to the work surface.
3. Coat a large bowl with cooking spray. Add the dough and turn it to coat with oil. Cover with a kitchen towel, set in a warm, draft-free place, and let the dough rise for 15 to 30 minutes.
4. Preheat the oven to 500°F.
5. Punch the dough down and cut it in half.
6. Lightly cover a work surface with flour. Begin rolling out the dough. When it starts to resist, roll it back into a ball and let it rest for several minutes.
7. Cover the work surface with more flour and roll out the dough again. When it resists or sticks to the surface, gather it back into a ball and let it rest for several minutes. Do this until the dough easily rolls into a 10-to-12-inch circle. It generally takes 4 times.
8. Carefully transfer the rolled pizza dough to a parchment-lined baking sheet without a rim. Add the desired amount of pizza sauce (I spread a thin layer), the preferred amount of cheese, and any desired toppings over the sauce.
9. Carefully slide the pizza crust (with the parchment paper—but without the baking sheet) onto the oven rack and cook for 5 to 7 minutes or until the cheese is bubbly and the edges of the crust are golden brown. Cut into wedges and serve immediately.

Embellishments

FLAVORED WHIPPED CREAM, GRANOLA, AND MISCELLANY

So much of what is in this chapter can be purchased ready-made, but those store-bought items don't compare to the taste of made-from-scratch. If anything, homemade is infinitely fresher, as well as prepared using wholesome ingredients without additives or chemicals.

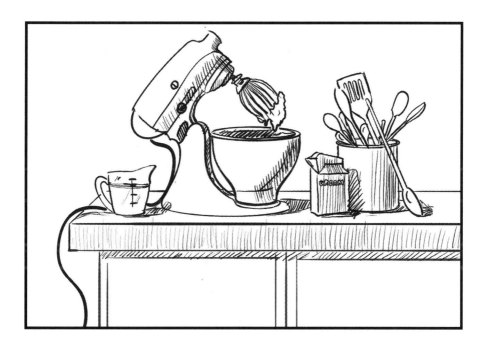

RECIPE INDEX

FLAVORED WHIPPED CREAM

Pineapple Rum Whipped Cream 139
Raspberry Almond Whipped Cream 140
Strawberry Amaretto Whipped Cream 141

GRANOLA

Apricot, Pistachio, and Coconut Granola 142
Four-Seed Granola with Molasses and Cranberries 143

MISCELLANY

Simple Buttermilk Crepes 144
Thai Basil Peanut Pesto 145
Herb Garlic Butter 146
Tamari Peanut Sauce with Toasted Sesame and Red Curry 147
Autumn Spice Blend 148
Toasted Pesto Crumbs 149
Gingered Cranberry Sauce 150

PINEAPPLE RUM WHIPPED CREAM

For optimum flavor, the pineapple should be ripe. I spread this cream over traditional biscuits and slices of baked ham. It also complements pork loin, pork chops, and pork tenderloin. For the cream to whip properly, chill the mixing bowl and/or the beaters in the freezer for about 2 hours before whipping the cream.

About 2 cups

1 tablespoon butter
¾ cup pineapple, finely chopped
1 tablespoon dark rum
½ cup heavy whipping cream

1. Melt the butter in a sauté pan over moderate heat. Sauté the pineapple until soft. Add the rum and stir to combine. Set aside.
2. In a medium bowl, beat the whipping cream on medium speed. When the cream thickens, increase the speed and continue to beat until the cream falls in large globs and stiff peaks have formed. Fold in the pineapple mixture and combine until well blended. Serve immediately or refrigerate until serving time.

RASPBERRY ALMOND WHIPPED CREAM

Dip a chocolate brownie into this decadent cream and you will be in creamy chocolate raspberry glory. It also makes a great topping for assorted summer fruit with a garnish of fresh spearmint or peppermint leaves. For the cream to whip properly, place the mixing bowl and/or beaters in the freezer for about 2 hours prior to preparing.

About 2 cups

1 cup heavy whipping cream
⅓ cup raspberry preserves
1 teaspoon almond extract (or more to taste)

1. Pour the whipping cream into a medium bowl and beat on medium speed. When the cream thickens, increase the speed and continue to beat until the cream falls in large globs and stiff peaks have formed.
2. Fold in the raspberry preserves and almond extract, and mix until well blended. Serve immediately or cover and refrigerate until serving time.

STRAWBERRY AMARETTO WHIPPED CREAM

This flavored cream is delicious spooned over a mixture of fresh seasonal fruit. For the cream to whip properly, place the mixing bowl and/or beaters in the freezer for about 2 hours prior to preparing.

About 2 cups

½ cup heavy whipping cream
½ cup mascarpone
⅓ cup strawberry preserves
2 tablespoons Amaretto liqueur

1. Pour the whipping cream into a medium bowl and beat on medium speed. When the mixture thickens, increase the speed and continue to beat until the cream falls in large globs and stiff peaks have formed.
2. Fold in the mascarpone, strawberry preserves, and Amaretto. Beat until fully blended. Serve immediately or cover and refrigerate until serving time.

APRICOT, PISTACHIO, AND COCONUT GRANOLA

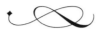

Granola is so satisfying. Delicious spooned over yogurt or ice cream, it can be added to cereal flakes and is a tasty topping for fresh seasonal fruit. One of my favorite discoveries is adding granola to leafy green salads; the naturally sweet granola is a flavorful replacement for savory bread croutons. The crunch factor of granola is a matter of preference; we like it very crispy and almost chestnut brown. This granola uses my recipe for autumn spice blend (see page 148). If you're not inclined to prepare the blend, you can substitute Spice Hunter's Winter Sippers Hot Buttered Rum Mix, available online.

About 4 cups

½ cup maple syrup
2 tablespoons neutral oil (expeller-pressed canola, high-oleic safflower, or
   sunflower oil)
2 tablespoons honey
3 tablespoons autumn spice blend
2 cups quick-cooking rolled oats
½ cup sliced almonds
½ cup sunflower seeds
½ cup shredded sweetened coconut
½ cup dried apricots, chopped
½ cup pistachios, chopped

1. Preheat the oven to 350°F.
2. Line the bottom of a rimmed baking sheet with parchment paper.
3. In a small pan, combine the maple syrup with the oil, honey, and autumn spice blend. Heat the mixture over moderate heat for 1 to 2 minutes.
4. Combine the oats with the almonds and sunflower seeds in a large bowl. Pour the maple mixture over the oat mixture and stir until evenly distributed. Transfer the mixture to the prepared baking sheet and spread the mixture in an even layer.
5. Bake for 12 to 18 minutes or until golden, stirring once halfway through the baking time. Allow the granola to cool. Once cooled, toss with coconut, apricots, and pistachios. Store the granola in an airtight container.

FOUR-SEED GRANOLA WITH MOLASSES AND CRANBERRIES

This recipe uses the autumn spice blend on page 148. If you're not inclined to prepare the blend, you can successfully substitute Spice Hunter's Winter Sippers Hot Buttered Rum Mix, available online.

About 3 cups

2 cups quick-cooking rolled oats
½ cup flaxseeds
½ cup sunflower seeds
¼ cup chia seeds
¼ cup sesame seeds
¼ cup neutral oil (expeller-pressed canola, high-oleic safflower, or sunflower oil)
¼ cup honey
¼ cup molasses
3 tablespoons autumn spice blend
½ teaspoon salt
½ teaspoon vanilla
½ cup dried cranberries

1. Preheat the oven to 350°F.
2. Line the bottom and sides of a rimmed baking sheet with parchment paper.
3. Combine the oats, flaxseeds, sunflower seeds, chia seeds, and sesame seeds in a large bowl.
4. In a small pan, combine the oil, honey, molasses, autumn spice blend, salt, and vanilla. Heat the mixture over moderate heat until warm. Pour the molasses mixture over the oat mixture and combine until evenly distributed.
5. Transfer the mixture to the prepared baking sheet and spread the mixture in an even layer. Bake for 18 to 20 minutes or until golden. Stir once halfway through the baking time. Allow the granola to cool slightly before tossing it with the cranberries. Store the granola in an airtight container.

SIMPLE
BUTTERMILK CREPES

Is there any other food that has as many possibilities as crepes? They can be eaten hot off the griddle with a slathering of anything savory or sweet, or they can be filled with just about any of your favorite food combinations and topped with a multitude of sauces. What's more, crepes can be served for breakfast, lunch, or dinner. Use your imagination for savory or sweet toppings and fillings. For added nutrition, color, and fun, add about 1 to 2 teaspoons of ground turmeric to the batter.

Here's a ridiculously simple crepe recipe that takes less than 5 minutes to prepare. I cook my crepes in a well-seasoned cast-iron skillet with a low lip. You really don't need a special pan to make a great crepe; any skillet with a shallow rim will work. Take note: It's best for the batter to sit refrigerated for about an hour. I love the rich flavor buttermilk gives to these crepes. If you don't have buttermilk on hand, whole milk works with the same results.

8 to 10 (8-inch) crepes

1¼ cups buttermilk
2 eggs
1 tablespoon butter, melted
¾ cup unbleached all-purpose flour
½ teaspoon salt
Butter for skillet

1. In a blender, or the bowl of a stand mixer, combine all the ingredients. Mix on medium-high speed until well blended. Let the batter rest for about 1 minute and blend again. Cover and refrigerate for about 1 hour.
2. Warm the skillet over moderately high heat and add a dollop of butter. When the butter has melted, add ¼ cup of the crepe batter and swirl the pan, allowing the batter to move nearly to the edge of the skillet. When the underside of the crepe is lightly brown, carefully flip the crepe, and cook for about 1 minute.
3. Cook the crepes in batches, adding more butter before adding crepe batter. If you're not cooking the crepes to order, transfer the cooked crepes to a pie plate, cover with a damp kitchen towel, and keep them warm in the oven set to the lowest temperature. Serve immediately.

THAI BASIL PEANUT PESTO

One year I planted Thai basil in my garden. The harvest was so plentiful, I found myself creating all sorts of uses for this basil. (The taste is very similar to that of traditional basil, but with a hint of lavender undertones.) It's delicious tossed with rice noodles, and Thai basil peanut pesto complements summer rolls.

1 cup Thai basil leaves
½ cup peanuts, roasted and salted
2 tablespoons grapeseed oil
2 tablespoons coconut butter
1 tablespoon rice vinegar
Salt, to taste (optional)

1. In a food processor, combine the basil leaves, peanuts, grapeseed oil, coconut butter, and vinegar. Pulse until the mixture is combined. If desired, season with salt to taste. Use immediately or transfer to a container, cover, and leave at room temperature until serving time. Refrigerate any unused portion.

HERB GARLIC BUTTER

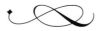

Who doesn't love bread slathered with garlic butter and then toasted until golden brown? In this recipe, I've added a little olive oil to the butter and several herbs. I briefly roast the garlic to soften the cloves. Roasting the cloves also removes the bitter flavor that is sometimes present in raw garlic. The amount of garlic is a matter of preference. For us, the more the better.

1 head of garlic (or about 15 to 20 cloves)
1 stick (½ cup) butter, softened
3 tablespoons olive oil
¼ teaspoon marjoram
¼ teaspoon oregano
¼ teaspoon rosemary
¼ teaspoon tarragon
¼ teaspoon thyme

1. Preheat the oven to 350°F.
2. Separate the garlic cloves, leaving the skin intact, and roast for 7 to 10 minutes or until soft. When the garlic is cool enough to handle, remove the skin and mince the cloves.
3. In a medium bowl, whisk the butter with the olive oil until well blended. Whisk in the marjoram, oregano, rosemary, tarragon, and thyme. Add the minced cloves and whisk until fully combined.
4. Generously spread the mixture on your favorite bread or refrigerate until serving time. If you refrigerate the butter, give the mixture a little time to soften slightly before spreading.

TAMARI PEANUT SAUCE WITH TOASTED SESAME AND RED CURRY

This sauce, with its lively flavor, complements baked chicken, tofu, and summer rolls. It is also a delicious dressing for buckwheat noodles.

½ cup tamari
1 tablespoon natural chunky peanut butter
1 tablespoon toasted sesame oil
½ teaspoon turmeric powder
1 teaspoon red curry paste
1 clove garlic, minced

1. In a medium bowl, whisk the tamari with the peanut butter, toasted sesame oil, turmeric, red curry paste, and garlic. Mix until well blended. Serve immediately or cover and keep at room temperature until serving time. Refrigerate any unused portion.

AUTUMN SPICE BLEND

This complementary blend transforms the flavor of ordinary muffin, waffle, and pancake batters. Truly a flavor enhancer, it is called for in many of the recipes in this cookbook. It is super-simple to put together and will keep for weeks if stored in an airtight container.

About 1 pound

1 pound light brown sugar
5 teaspoons cinnamon
4 teaspoons nutmeg
2 teaspoons ground cloves
2 teaspoons cardamom
1 teaspoon allspice
1 teaspoon lemon oil

1. In large bowl, combine the brown sugar with the spices. Toss the mixture until well blended. Add the lemon oil and toss until the ingredients are fully incorporated.
2. Transfer the mixture to an airtight container.

TOASTED PESTO CRUMBS

I love toasted pesto crumbs and use them all summer long—a complementary condiment I have on hand when basil is brimming in the garden. The crumbs are delicious accompanied by tomatoes (see recipe on page 89 for heirloom tomato and mozzarella salad). They are a great topping for pizza, summer casseroles, quiches, pasta, poached eggs, or anything that will benefit from a crunchy, flavorful, basil-infused topping. Leftover pesto will keep for weeks refrigerated, and you will have more pesto than what is called for in the toasted pesto crumbs recipe. For optimum flavor, I recommend making the bread crumbs from good-quality bread or homemade bread, rather than using store-bought bread crumbs.

About 1 cup

PESTO

> 2½ cups firmly packed fresh basil leaves
> 2 large garlic cloves
> ½ cup chopped almonds
> ½ cup freshly grated Parmesan cheese
> ½ cup olive oil
> Salt, to taste

1. Combine the basil leaves, garlic cloves, chopped almonds, and Parmesan cheese in a food processor fitted with a steel blade. Pulse a few times.
2. While the motor is running, drizzle the olive oil through the feed tube and whirl the mixture until well combined. Season with salt to taste. If you're not preparing the toasted pesto crumbs immediately, transfer the pesto to a container and refrigerate until serving.

TOASTED PESTO CRUMBS

> ⅔ cup dry bread crumbs
> ¼ cup pesto
> ⅛ cup olive oil

1. In a medium skillet over moderate heat, toast the crumbs until light brown.
2. Combine the bread crumbs with the pesto and olive oil in a small bowl. Stir until well combined.
3. If not using immediately, transfer to a container and cover until serving time.

GINGERED CRANBERRY SAUCE

This super-simple and tasty sauce is refreshingly delicious and a great complement to Thanksgiving turkey, but don't limit this sauce to the holidays. It's a terrific spread for chicken and/or turkey sandwiches and is beautiful spooned over vanilla or coconut ice cream. You can successfully prepare this in advance, and it will last for several days in the refrigerator. If you need a recommendation for ginger preserves, see the Product Reference Guide, page 233.

About 1 cup

12 ounces fresh cranberries, rinsed
½ cup ginger preserves

1. Combine the cranberries with the ginger preserves in a medium saucepan. Bring the mixture to a boil. Decrease the heat and cook for 5 to 10 minutes, stirring occasionally, until the cranberries pop open.
2. Once the sauce has cooled, transfer to a container, cover, and refrigerate until serving time.

Morning Meals

MUFFINS
PANCAKES, WAFFLES, AND FRENCH TOAST
COFFEE CAKES
SAVORY EGG DISHES

When my mother was in the kitchen, it seemed like the power of innovation was set into motion. Complementary and unusual combinations came to her easily. Breakfast was no exception, as she blended nutrient-rich ingredients like unusual grains—wheat germ and corn flour, for example—dried fruit, and nuts. Decades later, as I make batter for muffins, pancakes, and waffles, recalling her innovative creations gives me license, as well as confidence, to add formerly unlikely ingredients that are more commonly used now—chia, wheat germ, millet, spelt, quinoa, and ginger, and a broader variety of dried fruits such as apricots and cherries.

In this predominately vegetarian-inspired chapter, many of the recipes call for fruits available locally, while others suggest including fruits from around the globe. When fresh seasonal fruit is unavailable, I often rely on mangoes, bananas, pineapples, kiwi, pomegranate, citrus fruits, and coconut when they are in season in their native growing regions.

So, breakfast lovers, dive in. There is an abundance of nutrient-rich, savory, and sweet recipes to prepare in this chapter—six unique muffin recipes, recipes for pancakes, waffles, and French toast, four irresistible coffee cakes, and a selection of go-to egg dishes, including a few that are perfect to serve when hosting a crowd for brunch.

RECIPE INDEX

MUFFINS

Date and Apricot Muffins with Walnuts and Flaxseeds 154
Mango and Coconut Muffins 155
Chia-Cherry Muffins with Almonds and Millet 156
Pumpkin and Millet Muffins with Autumn Spice Blend 157-158
Quinoa Muffins with Flaxseed and Sunflower Seeds 159
Coconut Cherry Muffins with Pistachios 160

PANCAKES, WAFFLES, AND FRENCH TOAST

Gingered Mango Pancakes 161
Coconut Cottage Cheese Pancakes 162
Raspberry Pancakes 163
Quinoa Chia Pancakes 164
Oatmeal Chia Pancakes with Ginger Preserves 165
Cottage Cheese Pancakes 166
Pineapple Upside-Down Pancakes 167
Banana Upside-Down Pancakes 168
Coconut and Mango Lassi Pancakes 169
Mango Waffles 170
Blackened Banana Waffles 171
Cherry-and-Cream-Cheese-Stuffed French Toast 172

COFFEE CAKES

Raspberry Almond Coffee Cake with Almond Streusel 173-174
Pumpkin Coffee Cake with Crunchy Granola Topping 175
Peach and Cardamom Coffee Cake with Almond Butter Streusel 176-177
Pineapple and Cardamom Coffee Cake with Coconut Macadamia Streusel 178-179

SAVORY EGG DISHES

Fire-Roasted Tomato, Eggplant, Bacon, and Bean Casserole with Poached Eggs 180-181

Company Mushroom, Sausage, and Egg Casserole 182-183

Cauliflower and Roasted Red Pepper Quiche 184-185

Scrambled Eggs with Thyme 186

Poached Eggs over Couscous with a Pop of Harissa Heat 187-188

Mushroom and Spinach Brunch Casserole 189-190

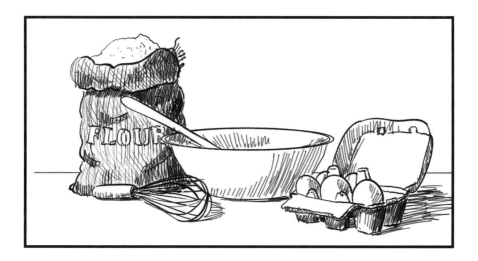

DATE AND APRICOT MUFFINS WITH WALNUTS AND FLAXSEED

When the leaves begin to change colors and the temperatures turn chilly, our appetites turn to heartier foods. It's around that time I make these autumn-inspired breakfast muffins.

12 muffins

1 cup unbleached all-purpose flour
1 cup walnuts, chopped
½ cup brown sugar
¼ cup wheat germ
¼ cup ground flaxseed
1 teaspoon salt
1 teaspoon baking soda
1 teaspoon baking powder
½ cup dates, chopped
½ cup dried apricots, chopped
1 egg
1¼ cups buttermilk
⅓ cup neutral oil (expeller-pressed canola, high-oleic safflower, or sunflower oil)

1. Preheat the oven to 350°F.
2. Generously oil a standard 12-capacity 2¾ x 1⅛-inch muffin pan with cooking spray.
3. Combine the flour, walnuts, brown sugar, wheat germ, ground flaxseed, salt, baking soda, and baking powder in a large bowl. Fold in the dates and apricots.
4. Whisk the egg with the buttermilk and oil in a medium bowl, and add to the flour mixture. Combine the ingredients until well blended.
5. Distribute the batter evenly into the prepared muffin pan compartments. Bake for 18 to 20 minutes or until a toothpick inserted in the center of a muffin comes out clean. Cool the muffins for 5 to 10 minutes before removing them from the muffin compartments.

MANGO AND COCONUT MUFFINS

Mango and coconut are the heroes in these delectable muffins, and, while they are perfectly delicious and moist on their own, we love to flood them with butter. For optimum flavor, the mango should be ripe. Alphonso mango, a personal favorite, is one of the most popular varieties because of its intense sweetness and rich flavor. For more about this mango variety, see the Product Reference Guide, page 233.

12 muffins

1⅓ cup unbleached all-purpose flour
⅓ cup corn flour
1 teaspoon baking soda
1 teaspoon baking powder
½ teaspoon salt
1 cup shredded sweetened coconut
2 eggs
6 ounces plain yogurt
⅓ cup neutral oil (expeller-pressed canola, high-oleic safflower, or sunflower oil)
1 teaspoon almond extract
1 cup mango, chopped
Butter

1. Preheat the oven to 350°F.
2. Generously oil a standard 12-capacity 2¾ x 1⅛-inch muffin pan with cooking spray.
3. Combine the flour, corn flour, baking soda, baking powder, salt, and coconut in a large bowl.
4. Lightly beat the eggs in a medium bowl. Add the yogurt, oil, and almond extract and stir until well blended. Add the egg mixture to the flour mixture. Combine the ingredients until well incorporated. Fold in the chopped mango.
5. Distribute the batter evenly into the muffin pan compartments. Bake for 12 to 15 minutes or until a toothpick inserted in the center of a muffin comes out clean. Cool the muffins for 5 to 10 minutes before removing them from the muffin compartments.

CHIA-CHERRY MUFFINS WITH ALMONDS AND MILLET

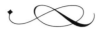

I love dried cherries, and they add a depth of flavor to these protein-packed, nutrient-rich muffins. To further enhance the multitude of flavors, spread the muffins with butter.

12 muffins

½ cup millet
1 cup whole wheat flour
1 cup almonds, chopped
½ cup corn flour
½ cup brown sugar
¼ cup chia seeds
1 teaspoon salt
1 teaspoon baking soda
1 egg
1¼ cups buttermilk
⅓ cup neutral oil (expeller-pressed canola, high-oleic safflower, or sunflower oil)
1 teaspoon almond extract
1 cup dried cherries, chopped
Butter, if desired

1. Preheat the oven to 350°F.
2. Place the millet on a rimmed baking sheet and bake for 10 to 12 minutes or until lightly browned and toasted. Watch closely; millet toasts very quickly.
3. Generously oil a standard 12-capacity 2¾ x 1⅛-inch muffin pan with cooking spray.
4. Combine the whole wheat flour, almonds, corn flour, toasted millet, brown sugar, chia seeds, salt, and baking soda in a large bowl.
5. Whisk the egg with the buttermilk, oil, and almond extract in a medium bowl. Add the liquid ingredients to the flour mixture and combine the ingredients until well blended. Fold in the cherries.
6. Distribute the batter evenly into the muffin pan compartments. Bake for 18 to 20 minutes or until a toothpick inserted in the center of a muffin comes out clean. Cool the muffins for 5 to 10 minutes before removing from muffin compartments.

Pumpkin and Millet Muffins with Autumn Spice Blend

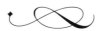

Toasted millet gives these muffins a wonderful crunch. Pure pumpkin gives them a pleasing cake-like texture. Served hot from the oven and slathered with butter, they are moist and decadent. Plan accordingly; this recipe uses the autumn spice blend on page 148. If you're not inclined to prepare the blend, Spice Hunter Hot Buttered Rum Mix, available online, is a fine replacement. Be sure to use real pumpkin and not pumpkin pie filling.

12 muffins

⅓ cup millet
1⅓ cups unbleached all-purpose flour
⅔ cup spelt flour
⅓ cup granulated sugar
⅓ cup autumn spice blend
1 teaspoon baking powder
½ teaspoon baking soda
½ teaspoon salt
1 egg
1 cup buttermilk
1 cup pure pumpkin
¼ cup neutral oil (expeller-pressed canola, high-oleic safflower, or sunflower oil)
Butter

1. Preheat the oven to 350°F.
2. Place the millet on a rimmed baking sheet and bake for 10 to 12 minutes, or until lightly browned and toasted. Watch closely; millet toasts very quickly.
3. Generously oil a standard 12-capacity 2¾ x 1⅛-inch muffin pan with cooking spray.
4. Combine the flour, spelt flour, sugar, autumn spice blend, toasted millet, baking powder, baking soda, and salt in a medium bowl.
5. Lightly beat the egg in a large bowl. Add the buttermilk, pumpkin, and oil, and stir until well blended. Add the flour mixture to the pumpkin mixture and combine until incorporated.

6. Distribute the batter evenly into the muffin pan compartments. Bake for 15 minutes or until a toothpick inserted in the center of a muffin comes out clean. Cool the muffins for 5 to 10 minutes before removing them from the muffin compartments.

Quinoa Muffins with Flaxseed and Sunflower Seeds

Rev up your weekday mornings with these protein-packed, nutrient-rich muffins.

12 muffins

½ cup water
⅓ cup plain quinoa
1 cup unbleached all-purpose flour
⅓ cup corn flour
⅓ cup spelt flour
⅓ cup brown sugar
¼ cup flaxseed, ground
1 teaspoon salt
1 teaspoon baking soda
2 eggs
½ cup milk
½ cup plain yogurt
½ cup neutral oil (expeller-pressed canola, high-oleic safflower, or sunflower oil)
½ cup raw sunflower seeds

1. Bring water to a boil in a small pan. Stir in the quinoa, remove from heat, cover, and set aside.
2. Preheat the oven to 350°F.
3. Generously oil a standard 12-capacity 2¾ x 1⅛-inch muffin pan with cooking spray.
4. Combine the flour, corn flour, spelt flour, brown sugar, ground flaxseed, salt, and baking soda in a large bowl.
5. Combine the eggs, milk, yogurt, and oil in a medium bowl. Add the liquid mixture to the flour mixture and combine until the ingredients are well blended. Fold in the quinoa and sunflower seeds and combine to distribute evenly.
6. Distribute the batter evenly into the muffin pan compartments. Bake for 12 to 15 minutes or until a toothpick inserted in the center of a muffin comes out clean. Cool the muffins for 5 to 10 minutes before removing them from the muffin compartments.

Coconut Cherry Muffins with Pistachios

I love the combination of coconut and cherries. The addition of pistachios give these nutrient-rich muffins a welcome crunch.

12 muffins

1 cup unbleached all-purpose flour
1 cup pistachios, chopped
¼ cup brown sugar
¼ cup wheat germ
¼ cup ground flaxseed
1 teaspoon salt
1 teaspoon baking soda
1 teaspoon baking powder
1 egg
1¼ cups buttermilk
⅓ cup neutral oil (expeller-pressed canola, high-oleic safflower, or sunflower oil)
1½ cups shredded sweetened coconut
½ cup dried cherries, chopped

1. Preheat the oven to 350°F.
2. Generously oil a standard 12-capacity 2¾ x 1⅛-inch muffin pan with cooking spray.
3. Combine the flour, pistachios, brown sugar, wheat germ, flaxseed, salt, baking soda, and baking powder in a large bowl.
4. Whisk the egg with the buttermilk and oil in a medium bowl. Add to the flour mixture and combine the ingredients until well blended. Fold in the coconut and cherries.
5. Distribute the batter evenly into the muffin pan compartments. Bake for 18 to 20 minutes or until a toothpick inserted in the center of a muffin comes out clean. Cool the muffins for 5 to 10 minutes before removing from the muffin compartments.

GINGERED MANGO PANCAKES

To me, ginger and mango go together like peanut butter and jelly. For optimal flavor, the mango should be ripe. For more about the best-tasting mangoes, visit the Product Reference Guide, page 233.

14 to 16 pancakes

1 cup ripe mango, diced
1 teaspoon ground ginger
1½ cups unbleached all-purpose flour
1½ teaspoons baking powder
½ teaspoon baking soda
½ teaspoon salt
2 eggs
1 cup milk
2 tablespoons neutral oil (expeller-pressed canola, high-oleic safflower, or
*   sunflower oil)*
1 teaspoon vanilla
Coconut oil for cooking pancakes
Butter and syrup

1. Toss the mango with the ginger in a medium bowl.
2. Combine the flour, baking powder, baking soda, and salt in a large bowl.
3. In a medium bowl, whisk the eggs, milk, oil, and vanilla until fully combined. Add the liquid mixture to the flour mixture and stir just to combine. Add the ginger/mango mixture.
4. Heat about 1 tablespoon of coconut oil in a large skillet over moderate heat. Spoon about ¼ cup of batter (per pancake) into the skillet; a large skillet will cook approximately 3 pancakes at a time. Cook pancakes for 1 or 2 minutes per side or until golden brown. Serve immediately with butter and syrup.

COCONUT COTTAGE CHEESE PANCAKES

If you're a coconut lover, you will love these pancakes. Coconut milk naturally separates and hardens—it will become fluid when heated. Shake the can well before opening and stir until fully blended before adding to the egg mixture.

About 2 dozen pancakes

2 eggs
2 tablespoons granulated sugar
2 tablespoons neutral oil (expeller-pressed canola, high-oleic safflower, or
    sunflower oil)
1 can (14 ounces) coconut milk
½ cup cottage cheese
1 cup shredded sweetened coconut, plus extra to garnish pancakes
1 cup unbleached all-purpose flour
¼ cup wheat germ
¼ cup spelt flour
3 teaspoons baking powder
½ teaspoon salt
Butter and syrup

1. Beat the eggs in a large bowl until well combined. Add the sugar and oil, and beat until light and fluffy. Add the coconut milk, shredded coconut, and cottage cheese and stir until well blended.

2. In a small bowl, combine the all-purpose flour, wheat germ, and spelt flour with the baking powder and salt. Add the flour mixture to the coconut mixture and combine until fully blended.

3. Heat about 1 tablespoon of oil in a large skillet over moderate heat. Spoon the batter into the skillet. A large skillet will cook approximately 3 pancakes at a time. Cook the pancakes for 1 or 2 minutes per side or until golden brown. Serve immediately with butter and syrup. Garnish the pancakes with shredded coconut.

RASPBERRY PANCAKES

Raspberries are one of the most delicate of all summer berries. Because they are highly perishable, they are best eaten shortly after they are purchased and/or harvested. Just before adding the berries to the pancake batter, gently wash the berries and place them on a paper towel. To remove any excess water that often gets caught in the opening of the berry, give them a gentle shake.

About 12 pancakes

¾ cup unbleached all-purpose flour
¼ cup wheat germ
2 teaspoons baking powder
1 tablespoon granulated sugar
⅛ teaspoon salt
1 egg
1 cup milk
1 teaspoon vanilla
1 cup raspberries, plus extra for garnishing pancakes
Butter, syrup, and confectioners' sugar

1. Combine the flour, wheat germ, baking powder, sugar, and salt in a large bowl.
2. Whisk the egg in a medium bowl. Add the milk and vanilla, and whisk until blended. Add 1 cup of raspberries and, using the tines of a serving fork, slightly mash them.
3. Add the liquid ingredients to the dry ingredients and stir until just combined.
4. Coat a large skillet with oil and heat over medium-high heat. Spoon or pour about ¼ cup of the batter into the skillet for each pancake; a large skillet cooks about 3 pancakes at a time. Cook for about 2 minutes on each side or until light brown. Garnish the pancakes with raspberries and dust with confectioners' sugar. Serve immediately with butter and syrup.

QUINOA CHIA PANCAKES

When I was creating the combination for these pancakes, I thought that maybe the quinoa and spelt flour would make them heavy. Not so. Happily, we found them amazingly light and fluffy. You can hardly detect a grain in these delicately flavored, nutritious, protein-rich breakfast pancakes. If you don't use all the batter at once, leftover batter will turn the color of chia seeds—grayish brown. A good stir will turn it back to the initial color.

14 to 16 pancakes

½ cup water
⅓ cup plain quinoa
2 eggs
2 tablespoons granulated sugar
2 tablespoons neutral oil (expeller-pressed canola, high-oleic safflower, or
    sunflower oil)
1½ cups buttermilk
1 tablespoon chia seeds
¾ cup unbleached all-purpose flour
¼ cup spelt flour
3 teaspoons baking powder
½ teaspoon salt
Butter and syrup

1. Boil the water in a small pan. Stir in the quinoa, remove from heat, cover, and set aside for 5 minutes.
2. Beat the eggs in a large bowl until well combined. Add the sugar and oil, and beat until light and fluffy. Add the buttermilk and chia seeds, and beat until well incorporated. Add the cooked quinoa and stir to combine.
3. Combine the flour, spelt flour, baking powder, and salt in a small bowl. Add the flour mixture to the quinoa mixture and combine until fully blended.
4. Heat about 1 tablespoon of oil in a large skillet over moderately high heat. Spoon or pour about ¼ cup of batter per pancake into the skillet; a large skillet will cook approximately 3 pancakes at a time. Cook pancakes for 1 or 2 minutes per side or until golden brown and the batter is cooked. Reduce the heat after you turn the pancakes to allow them to cook through and to keep them from burning. Serve immediately with butter and syrup.

OATMEAL CHIA PANCAKES WITH GINGER PRESERVES

Chia seeds give these nutrient-rich pancakes added crunch, and their mellow flavor is further enhanced by warmed ginger preserves. For my ginger preserve recommendation, see the Product Reference Guide, page 233. If you don't use all the batter at once, leftover batter will turn the color of chia seeds—grayish brown. A good stir will turn it back to the initial color. Ginger preserves have a pronounced flavor (can be overpowering for a young palate). Sample a spoonful on the pancakes, and then add the desired amount.

14 to 16 pancakes

2 eggs
2 tablespoons granulated sugar
2 tablespoons neutral oil (expeller-pressed canola, high-oleic safflower, or
    sunflower oil)
1½ cups buttermilk
1 cup quick-cooking oatmeal
½ cup unbleached all-purpose flour
¼ cup spelt flour
¼ cup whole wheat flour
1 tablespoon chia seeds
3 teaspoons baking powder
½ teaspoon salt
1 jar (12 ounces) ginger preserves
Butter

1. Beat the eggs in a large bowl until well combined. Add the sugar and oil, and beat until light and fluffy. Add the buttermilk and oatmeal, and combine until well blended.
2. Combine the flour, spelt flour, whole wheat flour, chia seeds, baking powder, and salt in a small bowl. Add the flour mixture to the oatmeal mixture and combine until fully blended.
3. Warm the ginger preserves in a small pan over low heat.
4. Heat about 1 tablespoon of oil in a large skillet over moderately high heat. Spoon or pour about ¼ cup of batter per pancake into the skillet; a large skillet will cook approximately 3 pancakes at a time. Cook the pancakes for 1 or 2 minutes per side or until golden brown and cooked through. Reduce the heat after you flip the pancakes to allow them to cook through and to keep them from burning. Serve immediately. Pass the warm ginger preserves and butter to your guests.

COTTAGE CHEESE PANCAKES

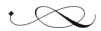

These surprisingly light, moist, tender, and fluffy pancakes have the added benefit of protein from the cottage cheese. Their flavor is further enhanced when they are topped with seasonal fruit. In the winter months, I sauté apples or pears in butter, season them with cinnamon, and top the pancakes with the warm fruit. Throughout the summer, I follow the fruit season and top the pancakes with the sweet bounty of unadorned berries and stone fruit.

4 servings

1 cup unbleached all-purpose flour
1 teaspoon baking soda
1 teaspoon baking powder
¼ teaspoon salt
2 tablespoons granulated sugar
3 eggs
1 cup cottage cheese
½ cup milk
2 tablespoons coconut oil
Butter and syrup
Seasonal fruit

1. Combine the flour, baking soda, baking powder, salt, and sugar in a medium bowl.
2. Whisk the eggs in a large bowl. Add the cottage cheese, milk, and oil, and stir until incorporated.
3. Add the flour mixture to the egg mixture and stir until completely blended.
4. Coat a large skillet with oil and heat over medium-high heat. Spoon about ¼ cup of the batter into the skillet for each pancake; a large skillet cooks about 3 pancakes at a time. Cook for about 2 minutes on each side or until light brown and cooked through. Serve immediately with butter and syrup. Top with fruit if desired.

PINEAPPLE UPSIDE-DOWN PANCAKES

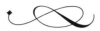

Nick likes these pancakes almost as much as he likes pineapple upside-down cake. For optimal flavor, the pineapple should be ripe.

6 to 8 pancakes

⅔ cup unbleached all-purpose flour
⅓ cup corn flour
⅓ cup wheat germ
1½ teaspoons baking powder
1½ teaspoons baking soda
½ teaspoon salt
1 cup buttermilk
1 egg
6-8 slices ripe pineapple
Butter and syrup

1. Combine the flour, corn flour, wheat germ, baking powder, baking soda, and salt in a large bowl.
2. Whisk the buttermilk with the egg yolk in a medium bowl.
3. Add the buttermilk/egg yolk mixture to the dry ingredients and stir using swift strokes.
4. In another medium bowl, beat the egg white until stiff peaks form. Fold the beaten egg white into the batter.
5. Generously coat a large skillet with oil and heat over medium-high heat. Spoon about ¼ cup of the batter into the skillet. The batter is thick, so spread it a little to accommodate the size of the pineapple slice. Add the pineapple slice. Lower the heat slightly and cook for approximately 2 minutes on each side or until cooked through and golden brown. Serve immediately with butter and syrup.

BANANA UPSIDE-DOWN PANCAKES

We enjoyed the pineapple upside-down pancakes so much (see page 167) that one morning I turned perfectly ripe bananas into banana upside-down pancakes and we loved them! Ripe bananas make these pancakes so creamy.

6 to 8 pancakes

⅔ cup unbleached all-purpose flour
⅓ cup corn flour
⅓ cup quick-cooking oatmeal
1½ teaspoons baking powder
1½ teaspoons baking soda
½ teaspoon salt
1 cup buttermilk
1 egg, separated
2 ripe bananas, sliced
Butter and syrup

1. Combine the flour, corn flour, oatmeal, baking powder, baking soda, and salt in a large bowl.
2. Whisk the buttermilk with the egg yolk in a medium bowl.
3. Add the buttermilk/egg yolk mixture to the dry ingredients and stir using swift strokes.
4. In another medium bowl, beat the egg white until stiff peaks form. Fold the beaten egg white mixture into the batter.
5. Generously coat a large skillet with oil and heat over medium-high heat. Spoon about ¼ cup of the batter per pancake into the skillet. The batter is thick, so spread it a little. Top the batter with 4 to 5 slices of banana for each pancake. Lower the heat slightly and cook for approximately 2 minutes on each side or until cooked through and golden brown. Serve immediately with butter and syrup.

COCONUT AND MANGO LASSI PANCAKES

If you're not familiar with it, lassi is a yogurt-based drink available in many flavors such as strawberry, blueberry, banana, and mango. Each fruit-filled lassi is creamy, with enough sweetness to balance out the little bit of yogurt tanginess. The flavor and texture are somewhere between a standard milk-based smoothie and kefir milk. I love the mango variety because it has a distinct mango flavor and a gorgeous deep orange color. One morning I decided to add lassi to pancake batter. Decadent doesn't accurately describe these pancakes. Lassi is available from most health-oriented grocery stores nationwide.

14 to 16 pancakes

2 eggs
2 tablespoons neutral oil (expeller-pressed canola, high-oleic safflower, or
sunflower oil)
1 cup mango lassi
½ cup buttermilk
1 cup shredded sweetened coconut
1 cup unbleached all-purpose flour
3 teaspoons baking powder
¼ teaspoon salt
Butter and syrup

1. Beat the eggs in a large bowl until well combined. Add the oil and beat until light and fluffy. Add the mango lassi and buttermilk, and beat until well combined. Add shredded coconut.
2. Combine the flour with the baking powder and salt in a small bowl. Add the flour mixture to the mango/coconut mixture and combine until fully blended.
3. Heat about 1 tablespoon of oil in a large skillet over moderate heat. Spoon or pour about ¼ cup of batter (per pancake) into the skillet; a large skillet cooks approximately 3 pancakes at a time. Cook the pancakes for 1 or 2 minutes per side or until golden brown. Serve immediately with butter and syrup.

MANGO WAFFLES

For optimum flavor, the mango should be ripe. For more information about the tastiest variety of mangoes, see the Product Reference Guide, page 233.

6 waffles

1 cup buttermilk
¼ cup sour cream
1¼ cups unbleached all-purpose flour
¼ cup whole wheat flour
1¼ teaspoons baking powder
1 teaspoon baking soda
¼ teaspoon salt
1 cup mango (about 1 medium), finely chopped
Butter and syrup

1. Preheat the waffle iron.
2. Combine the egg yolks, buttermilk, and sour cream in a medium bowl. Whisk until well blended.
3. Combine the flour, whole wheat flour, baking powder, baking soda, and salt in a large bowl. Add the egg mixture to the flour mixture and combine the mixture using swift strokes.
4. In a large bowl, beat the egg whites until stiff. Fold the egg whites into the egg/flour mixture and fold until just barely blended. (Any egg white showing through the batter is fine.)
5. Spoon about ¾ cup of the batter into the center of the hot waffle iron. Cook for about 4 minutes or until the light indicator on the waffle iron goes off, or the iron stops emitting steam. Serve immediately with butter and syrup.

BLACKENED BANANA WAFFLES

A complimentary bag of Red Fife (a nutty-flavored flour milled from organic Red Fife heritage wheat berries) from a Canadian wheat farmer prompted these waffles. The heat from the waffle iron slightly blackens the partially exposed bananas. If you can't get Red Fife, use whole wheat flour.

6 to 8 waffles

1 cup Red Fife wheat flour
½ cup unbleached all-purpose flour
¼ cup wheat germ
2 teaspoons baking powder
½ teaspoon salt
3 eggs, separated
½ cup neutral oil (expeller-pressed canola, high-oleic safflower, or sunflower oil)
1½ cups buttermilk
Ripe bananas, sliced (about 8 thin slices per waffle)
Butter and syrup

1. Preheat the waffle iron.
2. Combine the Red Fife flour, all-purpose flour, wheat germ, baking powder, and salt in a large bowl.
3. Combine the egg yolks, oil, and buttermilk in a medium bowl. Add the egg mixture to the flour mixture and combine using swift strokes.
4. In a large bowl, beat the egg whites until stiff. Fold the egg whites into the waffle batter.
5. Spoon a heaping ½ cup of the batter into the center of the hot waffle iron. Spread the batter, using a rubber spatula, a little toward the edge (not too much, as the weight from the top of the waffle iron will distribute the batter). Lay the banana slices on top of the batter, about two slices per wedge. Cook for about 4 minutes or until the light indicator on the waffle iron goes off, or until the iron stops emitting steam. Serve immediately with butter and syrup.

CHERRY-AND-CREAM-CHEESE-STUFFED FRENCH TOAST

When cherries are in season, I love to serve this delicious dish when we're entertaining another couple for a morning meal. Not only is it impressive, I especially like that it must be prepared the day before you plan to serve it. More time to spend with guests! Pork sausage, vegetarian sausage, or bacon can be served as complementary accompaniments.

4 servings

4 ounces (block-style) ⅓ less fat cream cheese, at room temperature
1 cup dark cherries, pitted and chopped
1 tablespoon fresh lemon juice
8 slices (½ inch each) Tuscan or country-style white bread
4 eggs
½ cup half-and-half
1 to 2 tablespoons coconut oil
Confectioners' sugar (garnish)
Butter and syrup

1. Combine the cream cheese with the cherries in a small bowl.
2. Spread the cream cheese mixture evenly over four slices of bread. Top each prepared slice of bread with the remaining slices of bread.
3. In a baking dish that will accommodate 4 sandwiches in a single layer, whisk the eggs with the half-and-half. Place the sandwiches in the egg mixture and allow one side to soak in the egg mixture for 2 to 3 minutes, and then turn the sandwiches over. Cover and refrigerate overnight.
4. Prior to cooking, allow the French toast sandwiches to reach room temperature (about 30 minutes).
5. Heat the oil in a large skillet over moderately high heat, and cook the sandwiches (in batches of two, or in two skillets) until golden brown on each side. Transfer to serving plates and dust the French toast sandwiches with confectioners' sugar. Pass the butter and syrup to your guests.

RASPBERRY ALMOND COFFEE CAKE WITH ALMOND STREUSEL

Lactose-intolerant guests prompted the creation of this moist and delicious coffee cake. In winter, I yearn for summer fruit, particularly berries. The high quality of the Oregon line of canned fruit products satisfies on many levels. They can be found in most health-oriented grocery stores nationwide or online. After many attempts at testing almond milk, Califia Farms brand is my favorite; it has a rich almond flavor. It's also the only brand I found that was carrageenan-free.

8 servings

1 cup unbleached all-purpose flour
½ cup granulated sugar
1 teaspoon baking powder
½ teaspoon salt
¼ teaspoon baking soda
1 can (15 ounces) raspberries, drained
1 egg
⅔ cup almond milk
2 tablespoons neutral oil (expeller-pressed canola, high-oleic safflower, or
   sunflower oil)
½ teaspoon almond extract
2 tablespoons brown sugar
2 tablespoons unbleached all-purpose flour
¼ teaspoon cinnamon
2 tablespoons butter, cut into chunks
⅓ cup sliced almonds
Butter

1. Preheat the oven to 350°F.
2. Coat an 8 x 8 x 2-inch square baking pan with cooking spray.
3. Combine 1 cup of the flour, granulated sugar, baking powder, salt, and baking soda in a large bowl. Toss the flour mixture with half of the raspberries.

4. Combine the egg with the almond milk, oil, and almond extract in a medium bowl, and whisk until well blended. Pour the liquid mixture into the flour/raspberry mixture and stir until well incorporated. Transfer the batter into the prepared baking pan and top the mixture with the remaining raspberries.

5. Combine the brown sugar, 2 tablespoons of flour, and cinnamon in a small bowl. Add the chunks of butter and blend using your fingers until the mixture crumbles—this is the streusel. Distribute the butter mixture evenly over the cake batter and top the streusel mixture with the almonds. Bake for 35 minutes or until a toothpick inserted in the center of the cake comes out clean. Serve immediately with butter.

PUMPKIN COFFEE CAKE WITH CRUNCHY GRANOLA TOPPING

Like most coffee cakes, this tastes best eaten hot from the oven. Spreading it with butter is an option I enthusiastically endorse. I love to prepare this in the autumn months, and especially during Thanksgiving week when we are hosting family and friends. Make certain to purchase pure pumpkin and not pumpkin pie filling. Autumn-like, flavor-fused granola is a complementing choice.

6 servings

¾ cup unbleached all-purpose flour
¼ cup flaxseed, ground
½ cup granulated sugar
1 teaspoon baking powder
½ teaspoon salt
¼ teaspoon baking soda
1 egg
1 cup pure pumpkin
⅔ cup buttermilk
2 tablespoons neutral oil (expeller-pressed canola, high-oleic safflower, or sunflower oil)
¾ cup granola
2 tablespoons butter, cut into chunks
Butter, optional

1. Preheat the oven to 350°F.
2. Coat an 8 x 8 x 2-inch square baking pan with cooking spray.
3. Combine the flour, ground flaxseed, sugar, baking powder, salt, and baking soda in a large bowl.
4. Beat the egg in a medium bowl. Add the buttermilk and oil, and whisk until blended. Add the pumpkin and combine until fully incorporated. Add the pumpkin mixture to the flour mixture and stir until well incorporated.
5. Transfer the batter into the prepared baking pan. Distribute the granola evenly over the coffee cake batter. Dot the top with chunks of butter.
6. Bake for 35 minutes or until a toothpick inserted in the center of the cake comes out clean. Serve immediately. Pass the butter to your guests if desired.

PEACH AND CARDAMOM COFFEE CAKE WITH ALMOND BUTTER STREUSEL

This is an incredibly moist coffee cake with a wonderful fresh peach flavor, punctuated with just the right amount of aromatic cardamom. It needs nothing more than good company and a steaming cup of coffee or tea. The best time to prepare this coffee cake is when the peach orchard is brimming with its beautiful bounty.

6 servings

1 cup unbleached all-purpose flour
½ cup granulated sugar
¾ teaspoon baking powder
¼ teaspoon salt
¼ teaspoon baking soda
½ teaspoon cardamom
1¼ cups peaches, peeled and chopped
⅔ cup milk
2 tablespoons neutral oil (expeller-pressed canola, high-oleic safflower, or
    sunflower oil)
1 teaspoon vanilla
1 egg
¼ cup sliced almonds
1 tablespoon brown sugar
¼ teaspoon cinnamon
2 tablespoons butter

1. Preheat the oven to 350°F.
2. Coat an 8 x 8 x 2-inch square baking pan with cooking spray.
3. Combine the flour, sugar, baking powder, salt, baking soda, cardamom, and ¾ cup of the peaches in a large bowl. Toss well.
4. Combine the milk, oil, vanilla, and egg in a medium bowl, and whisk until well blended. Add the liquid mixture to the flour mixture and stir until well combined. Transfer the coffee cake to the prepared pan and top with the remaining chopped peaches.

5. Combine the almonds, brown sugar, cinnamon, and melted butter in a small bowl and then evenly distribute over the coffee cake.

6. Bake for 35 minutes or until a toothpick inserted in the center of the cake comes out clean. Serve immediately.

PINEAPPLE AND CARDAMOM COFFEE CAKE WITH COCONUT MACADAMIA STREUSEL

For optimum flavor, the pineapple should be ripe. Serve this globally inspired coffee cake warm from the oven and watch it disappear!

8 servings

1½ cups unbleached all-purpose flour
½ cup granulated sugar
2 teaspoons baking powder
½ teaspoon baking soda
½ teaspoon cardamom
¼ teaspoon salt
1 cup sour cream
2 eggs
1 cup ripe pineapple, chopped
2 tablespoons unbleached all-purpose flour
¼ cup granulated sugar
2 tablespoons butter, cut into chunks
¼ cup shredded sweetened coconut
¼ cup macadamia nuts, chopped

1. Preheat the oven to 350°F.
2. Coat an 8 x 8 x 2-inch square baking pan with cooking spray.
3. Combine 1½ cups of flour, ½ cup of sugar, baking powder, baking soda, cardamom, and salt in a large bowl.
4. Whisk the sour cream with the eggs in a medium bowl until well blended. Add the pineapple to the sour cream mixture. Add the pineapple/sour cream mixture to the flour mixture and stir until fully incorporated. Transfer the batter to the prepared pan.
5. Combine 2 tablespoons of the flour and ¼ cup of sugar in a small bowl. Add the chunks of butter and blend the mixture using your fingers until the mixture crumbles—this is

the streusel. Add the coconut to the butter mixture and mix until incorporated. Sprinkle the mixture evenly over the cake. Top with the chopped macadamia nuts. Bake for 35 to 40 minutes or until a toothpick inserted in the center of the cake comes out clean. Serve immediately.

Fire-Roasted Tomato, Eggplant, Bacon, and Bean Casserole with Poached Eggs

The cast-iron honey-glazed cornbread recipe on page 115 is a complementary accompaniment to this wholesome meal-in-one-dish. Don't limit this dish to breakfast or brunch fare; it's weeknight-friendly as well.

6 servings

1 medium eggplant, cut into ½-inch slices
Olive oil
Coarse salt
1 pound bacon
1 tablespoon neutral oil (expeller-pressed canola, high-oleic safflower, or sunflower oil)
4 cloves garlic, sliced
1 pound fresh spinach
1 can (28 ounces) fire-roasted tomatoes
1 can (15 ounces) black beans, drained
½ cup freshly grated Asiago cheese
1 cup freshly grated cheddar cheese
2 tablespoons apple cider vinegar
6 eggs

1. Preheat the oven to 350°F.
2. Place the eggplant slices on a parchment-lined rimmed baking sheet and brush them with olive oil. Season the slices with coarse salt and cook for a half hour or until fork-tender. When the eggplant is cool enough to handle, cut into cubes. Set aside.
3. While the eggplant is cooking, cook the bacon until crispy. When it's cool enough to handle, crumble. Set aside.
4. Heat the oil in a large pot over moderate heat and sauté the garlic for a few minutes. Add the spinach, reduce the heat, cover, and cook until the spinach has wilted. Transfer the spinach and garlic to a bowl. Set aside.

5. Spread half of the tomatoes in the bottom of an 11 x 7 x 2-inch baking dish. Top the tomatoes with the cubed eggplant and ¼ cup of Asiago cheese. Top the cheese with the spinach, black beans, and the remaining Asiago cheese. Top the cheese with the remaining tomatoes, crumbled bacon, and cheddar cheese. Cover and cook for 30 minutes or until bubbly. Remove the cover and cook for an additional 10 to 15 minutes.

6. While the dish is in the oven, fill a 2-quart pot with 1½ quarts of water. Bring the water to a boil. Add the vinegar. Reduce the heat to medium high (water should be actively rumbling, but not boiling). Break each egg into a small cup and gently slide each egg into the rumbling water. Working quickly, repeat with the remaining eggs. Cook the eggs for 3 to 5 minutes or until desired doneness. (For me, a perfectly cooked poached egg is when the white is hard and the yolk is runny.)

7. Divide the casserole between 6 rimmed serving dishes and top each with a poached egg. Serve immediately.

COMPANY MUSHROOM, SAUSAGE, AND EGG CASEROLE

This crowd-pleasing, piquant company brunch casserole always receives rave reviews because it's got many of the complementary breakfast ingredients people enjoy all in one dish. Taste-testers' favorite pairings were slices of fresh summer tomatoes or a tomato dish of any kind, and a seasonal fruit medley. For my vegetarian clients and friends, I've successfully made this using vegan sausage. Plan accordingly; this takes time to put together. You can prepare the mushroom mixture in advance, and you can precook the sausage. Allow them to come to room temperature before assembling with the rest of the ingredients.

14 servings

4 tablespoons butter
2 packages (8 ounces each) white mushrooms, chopped
2 tablespoons unbleached all-purpose flour
⅓ cup cooking sherry
1 teaspoon salt
A few grindings of black pepper
5 cups bread, cubed, and crusts removed
1 pound vegan or ground pork sausage, cooked
1½ cups cheddar cheese, shredded
1½ dozen eggs
3 cups milk
1½ teaspoons thyme
1 teaspoon dry mustard
1½ teaspoons salt

1. Melt the butter in a large skillet over moderate heat. Add the mushrooms and cook, stirring occasionally, for 5 minutes or until the mushrooms are tender. Sprinkle the flour over the mushrooms, and stir until they have grabbed all the flour. Reduce the heat to low and add the cooking sherry. Season the mushrooms with salt and pepper. Stir until the ingredients are well incorporated. Remove the skillet from the heat and set aside. (Don't worry about the mixture being thick.)
2. Coat the bottom and sides of a glass 15 x 10 x 2-inch baking dish with cooking spray.

3. Place the bread cubes in the baking dish and top with the sausage. Distribute the cheese over the sausage/bread mixture.

4. Preheat the oven to 350°F.

5. Whisk the eggs in a large bowl until well combined. Add the milk, thyme, dry mustard, and salt. Season with a few grindings of black pepper. Whisk until well incorporated. Pour the egg mixture over the bread/sausage/cheese mixture. Spoon the mushroom mixture over the eggs. (It doesn't have to be evenly distributed; it will spread while it's baking.) Bake for 30 to 35 minutes or until light brown. Serve immediately.

CAULIFLOWER AND ROASTED RED PEPPER QUICHE

This is a colorful, delicious combination I like to serve when hosting brunch. A fresh fruit medley or a tossed green salad rounds out this desirable meal. If time is of the essence, use a good-quality store-bought piecrust. Wholly Wholesome makes a close-to-homemade organic pie shell. In this recipe, jarred roasted red bell peppers are used.

6 servings

1¼ cups unbleached all-purpose flour
½ teaspoon salt
⅓ cup neutral oil (expeller-pressed canola, high-oleic safflower, or sunflower oil)
2½ to 3 tablespoons cold water
2 cups cauliflower pieces
8 eggs
½ cup half-and-half
½ teaspoon salt
½ teaspoon oregano
½ teaspoon marjoram
½ teaspoon thyme
A dash of cayenne pepper
1 tablespoon Dijon-style mustard
3 cups cheddar cheese, shredded
½ cup roasted red bell peppers, chopped

1. Combine the flour and salt in a medium bowl. Drizzle the oil over the flour and toss until the flour mixture is coarse. Slowly drizzle in the cold water. Add more water if the dough doesn't come together or seems dry. Knead the dough a few times to fully incorporate the ingredients. Let the dough rest for about 5 minutes.
2. Lightly flour a work surface and roll the dough until it's about 12 inches in diameter. If it resists, let it rest for about 5 minutes. Transfer to a 9-inch pie plate and flute the edges. Set aside.
3. Fill a large pot with a few inches of water and place a steamer basket on top—the water should be just below the holes of the steamer. Cover the pot and bring the water to a

boil. When the water has boiled, steam the cauliflower for 7 to 10 minutes or until just fork-tender. Remove the cauliflower from the steamer and set aside.

4. Preheat the oven to 350°F.

5. In a large bowl, whisk the eggs with the half-and-half, salt, oregano, marjoram, thyme, and cayenne pepper.

6. Evenly spread the mustard over the bottom of the unbaked pie shell. Sprinkle 1 cup of shredded cheese over the mustard. Top the cheese with 1 cup of cooked cauliflower and ¼ cup of chopped roasted red peppers. Top the mixture with 1 cup of cheese. Top the cheese with the remaining cauliflower and the roasted red pepper. Pour the egg mixture evenly over the cauliflower/roasted red pepper mixture and top with the remaining cheese. Bake for 45 minutes. Allow the quiche to sit for about 10 minutes before serving.

SCRAMBLED EGGS WITH THYME

Whenever my mother scrambled eggs, she always added a little bit of thyme. There was something so satisfying about the combination. I enjoy thyme's earthy flavor in eggs (and especially the aroma) as much now as I did when I first ate them as a child.

6 servings

12 eggs
3 tablespoons butter
1 teaspoon dried thyme
Salt and pepper, to taste

1. Whisk the eggs in a large bowl until well blended.
2. Melt the butter in a large skillet over moderate heat. Add the eggs. Allow the eggs to cook briefly undisturbed until a few bubbles appear. Sprinkle the thyme evenly over the eggs. Slowly drag a spatula across the bottom of the skillet, going from one side of the skillet to the other using a back-and-forth motion. Let the eggs sit undisturbed again for a few seconds. Drag the spatula again across the bottom of the skillet. Continue the dragging process at a more rapid pace. When the eggs begin to set, continue dragging the spatula and begin folding the eggs over themselves. When they are still a bit wet looking, remove the skillet from the heat. Transfer to serving plates and season with salt and pepper. Serve immediately.

POACHED EGGS OVER COUSCOUS WITH A POP OF HARISSA HEAT

One night while driving home from jury duty, rain pounding the windshield, desperately trying not to think about the day's events in court, I passed a restaurant Nick and I have enjoyed over the years. I reminisced about the unusual dish I often ordered when we ate there for breakfast. It was a perfectly cooked egg (white hard—yellow runny) that lay in the center of a mound of steamy, fluffy white rice that was topped with a spicy, vibrant red sauce. Thoughts of it made my mouth water. I set out to duplicate it the following day using couscous instead of rice and garnishing the eggs with olives, roasted red peppers, and harissa. It was a flavor sensation. Harissa is very spicy. Use it sparingly (or cut the amount of cayenne pepper in half) until you become familiar with its aftereffects. Jarred roasted red bell peppers can be found in the condiment aisle of most grocery stores. To make certain everyone gets their meal while it's still hot, warm the rimmed serving dishes.

6 servings

HARISSA

> *½ cup olive oil*
> *1 teaspoon cayenne pepper*
> *2 tablespoons tomato paste*
> *¼ cup fresh lime juice (about 1 medium lime)*
> *½ teaspoon salt*

1. Combine the olive oil, cayenne pepper, tomato paste, lime juice, and salt in a small bowl. Whisk until the mixture is emulsified. Set aside. (The olive oil naturally separates from the other ingredients; whisk just before serving.)

POACHED EGGS OVER COUSCOUS

> *1 box (10 ounces) plain couscous*
> *⅓ cup minced fresh parsley*
> *2 tablespoons apple cider vinegar*
> *6 eggs*
> *Kalamata black olives, pitted and chopped (garnish)*
> *Roasted red bell peppers, chopped (garnish)*

187

1. Fill a 2-quart pot with 1½ quarts of water. Bring the water to a boil.
2. While you are waiting for the water to boil, cook the couscous according to the package directions. Add the parsley and fluff the couscous to incorporate the parsley. Cover and keep warm.
3. When the water has boiled, add the vinegar and reduce the heat to medium high. (The water should be actively rumbling, but not boiling.) Break each egg into a small cup and gently slide each one into the rumbling water. Cook the eggs for 3 to 5 minutes or until desired doneness. (For me, a perfectly cooked poached egg is when the white is hard and the yolk is runny.)
4. Just before the eggs have finished cooking, divide the couscous among 6 rimmed serving dishes. Remove the eggs with a slotted spoon, drain them of any excess water, and place an egg on top of the couscous. Top with the desired amount of chopped olives and roasted red peppers. Serve immediately. Pass the spicy harissa to your guests.

MUSHROOM AND SPINACH BRUNCH CASSEROLE

This is very similar to the recipe for company mushroom, sausage, and egg casserole (see page 182). In this recipe, I swapped spinach for the sausage with wonderful results. Taste-testers' favorite pairings are a tomato dish, assorted fresh fruit, and slices of ham, crispy bacon, or sausage.

10 to 12 servings

3 tablespoons butter
1 package (10 ounces) or about 13 to 15 medium-sized white mushrooms, chopped
1 tablespoon flour
¼ cup cooking sherry
½ teaspoon salt
A few grindings of black pepper
4 cups bread with crust, cubed (good-quality Italian or French works well)
16 ounces frozen chopped spinach, defrosted, drained, and squeezed dry
1 cup shredded cheddar cheese
12 eggs
2 cups milk
1 teaspoon thyme
1 teaspoon salt
½ teaspoon dry mustard

1. Place the butter in a large skillet and melt over moderate heat. Add the mushrooms and cook until tender, about 5 minutes, stirring occasionally. Add the flour (the liquid from the mushrooms will grab the flour very quickly), and stir until fully combined. Remove the skillet from the heat and add the sherry, salt, and pepper. Stir until the ingredients are incorporated.
2. Preheat the oven to 350°F.
3. Place the bread cubes in a glass 13 x 9 x 2-inch baking dish. Top the bread cubes with the spinach (don't worry if the spinach doesn't cover the bread cubes evenly—it sorts itself out during the cooking process), and top with the shredded cheese.
4. Whisk the eggs in a large bowl until lightly beaten. Add the milk, thyme, salt, and dry mustard. Season with a few grindings of black pepper and whisk until well combined. Pour the egg mixture over the bread/spinach/cheese combination. Dot the top of the

casserole with the mushroom mixture. (The mushroom mixture won't cover the eggs; it will distribute more evenly when baking.) Bake uncovered for 1 hour. Serve immediately.

The Grand Finale

CAKES
ROLLED CAKES
PIES
COOKIES
ICE CREAM, AND DESSERT SOUP

This chapter brims with cakes, rolled cakes, pies, cookies, ice cream, and dessert soup—sweets that evoke childhood memories of birthday celebrations and other special occasions. Each brings back memories of favorite times gone by. I can't bake a cake without thinking about my mother's cakes; they were sometimes a bit lopsided, but always delicious.

Once a catering client asked me for a rolled cake. Since I had never made one, I tried to dissuade her, without success. After I created it, however, I was amazed at how easy it was and impressed with the outcome—as was my client. Once sliced, a rolled cake resembles a beautiful pinwheel. Soon I was "on a roll" creating roll cake recipes, and I encourage you to try at least one of the four included here.

For caramel and chocolate lovers, I've included my recipe for caramel chocolate pie with salty pretzel crust—so delicious that I created another recipe using whipped cream in place of chocolate. If you're a rhubarb fan, don't miss the rhubarb pie; rhubarb season is short and slips by quickly. An assorted variety of cookie recipes for the cookie basket and summery ice cream recipes—frozen margarita martinis with salty pretzel crust, coconut and roasted peanut ice cream with Thai basil, and the light and refreshing creamy strawberry soup with Amaretto—round out the selections in this eclectic chapter.

RECIPE INDEX

CAKES
Chocolate Cupcakes with Chocolate Pecan Icing 194-195
Chocolate Pomegranate Wine Cake 196
Date and Autumn Spice Cake 197
Mardi Gras Sugar-Glazed King Pastry Cake 198-199
Cardamom-Infused Cranberry Cobbler Cake 200-201
Fresh Strawberry Cake 202
Lemon and Ricotta Apple Cake 203
Apricot Chia Cake 204
Clove-Spiked Red Plum Cake 205

ROLLED CAKES
Strawberry-and-Cream-Filled Rolled Cake 206-207
Chocolate-and-Caramel-Filled Rolled Cake 208-209
Peaches-and-Cream-Filled Rolled Cake 210-211
Chocolate-Coconut-and-Gingered-Cranberry-Cream-Filled Rolled Cake 212-213

PIES
Caramel Chocolate Pie with Salty Pretzel Crust 214-215
Caramel Cream Pie with Salty Pretzel Crust 216-217
Chocolate, Coconut, and Peanut Butter Pie 218
Coconut Custard Pie 219
Rhubarb Pie 220-221

COOKIES

Bittersweet Chocolate Cookies with Sea Salt 222-223

Chocolate Fudge and Pistachio Nut Cookies 224

Lemon Crinkle Cookies 225

Almond Lace Cookies 226

Almond Cookies 227

ICE CREAM, AND DESSERT SOUP

Frozen Margarita Martinis with Salty Pretzel Crust 228-229

Coconut and Roasted Peanut Ice Cream with Thai Basil 230

Creamy Strawberry Soup with Amaretto 231

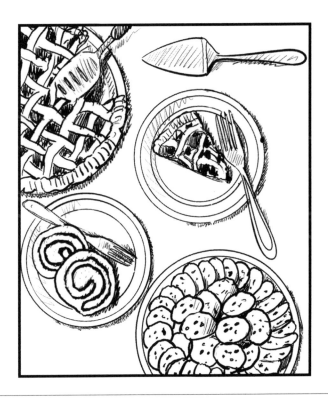

CHOCOLATE CUPCAKES WITH CHOCOLATE PECAN ICING

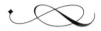

I can taste the flavors of my childhood in these rich and buttery chocolate-charged cupcakes. This moist cupcake always receives enthusiastic reviews. If you don't have buttermilk on hand, add 1 teaspoon of lemon juice or white vinegar to a half-cup of milk, and let the mixture stand for about 5 minutes.

24 cupcakes

2 cups unbleached all-purpose flour
2 cups granulated sugar
4 tablespoons cocoa powder
1 teaspoon baking soda
1 cup (2 sticks) butter
½ cup canola oil
1 cup water
2 eggs
½ cup buttermilk
1 teaspoon vanilla
2 tablespoons cocoa powder
6 tablespoons milk
1 box confectioners' sugar
1 teaspoon vanilla
1 cup pecans, chopped
2 dozen standard (2-inch x 1¼-inch) baking cup liners

1. Preheat the oven to 350°F.
2. Combine the flour, sugar, cocoa powder, and baking soda in a large bowl.
3. Melt 1 stick of butter and oil in a medium saucepan over moderate heat. Add the water and bring the mixture to a boil. Add to the dry ingredients and mix until well combined.
4. Whisk the eggs in a medium bowl until well combined. Add the buttermilk and vanilla. Add the buttermilk/egg mixture to the remaining ingredients and stir until fully combined. Fill the paper cupcake liners ¾ full and bake for 15 minutes or until a toothpick inserted in the center of a cupcake comes out clean.

5. Melt the remaining stick of butter in a large saucepan over low heat. Add cocoa powder and milk, and then whisk until well blended. Remove from heat and stir in the confectioners' sugar, vanilla, and pecans. Mix until well blended.

6. When the cupcakes have cooled, spread icing evenly over each cupcake.

CHOCOLATE POMEGRANATE WINE CAKE

During the Christmas holidays, one of our neighbors brought pomegranate wine to a neighborhood celebration. I added the leftover wine to chocolate cake batter, and, although the pomegranate flavor came through in a mellow way, taste-testers enjoyed the cake.

6 to 8 servings

1 cup granulated sugar
¾ cup unbleached all-purpose flour
⅓ cup cocoa powder
1 teaspoon baking soda
½ teaspoon baking powder
½ teaspoon salt
1 egg
½ cup buttermilk
½ cup pomegranate wine
¼ cup canola oil
1 teaspoon vanilla
Confectioners' sugar for dusting the top of the cake

1. Preheat the oven to 350°F.
2. Generously oil an 8 x 1½-inch round cake pan with cooking spray.
3. Combine the sugar, flour, cocoa, baking soda, and baking powder in a large bowl. Add the egg, buttermilk, wine, oil, and vanilla, and beat on medium speed until all the dry ingredients are incorporated.
4. Pour the batter into the prepared pan. Bake for 35 minutes or until a toothpick inserted in the center of the cake comes out clean.
5. Place the cake pan on a wire rack. When the cake is cool enough to handle, run a knife around the edge of the pan and carefully invert the cake onto a wire rack. Allow the cake to cool completely before transferring to a serving platter. Just before serving, dust the top with confectioners' sugar.

DATE AND AUTUMN SPICE CAKE

The combination of naturally sweet dates and the zesty flavors that come from the autumn spice blend (brown sugar, cinnamon, nutmeg, cardamom, allspice, cloves, and lemon oil) is what makes this rustic-looking, chestnut-colored cake packed with such dynamic flavor. If you're not inclined to prepare the blend (see page 148), Spice Hunter Hot Buttered Rum Mix, available online, is a fine replacement.

6 to 8 servings

½ cup canola oil
¾ cup granulated sugar
¼ cup autumn spice blend
2 eggs
1¼ cups unbleached all-purpose flour
1 tablespoon baking powder
¼ teaspoon salt
1 cup sour cream
1 cup dates, pitted and chopped
Confectioners' sugar for dusting the top of the cake

1. Preheat the oven to 400°F.
2. Generously oil a 9 x 1½-inch cake pan with cooking spray, and then dust the pan with flour.
3. Beat the canola oil in a large bowl on medium speed, and slowly add the sugar and autumn spice blend. Beat until light and fluffy. Lower the speed and add the eggs one at a time, beating well after each addition. Add the flour, baking powder, and salt, and beat until well blended. Add the sour cream and dates, and incorporate until well blended.
4. Transfer the batter to the prepared cake pan and bake for 35 minutes or until a toothpick inserted in the center of the cake comes out clean.
5. Allow the cake to cool before transferring to a serving platter. Just before serving, dust the top with confectioners' sugar.

MARDI GRAS SUGAR-GLAZED KING PASTRY CAKE

In case you're not familiar with it, king cake is not at all like a cake, but much more like a rolled pastry; hence the name, king pastry cake. The cake traditionally includes a token. Whoever gets the token in their piece of cake is the next person to host a Mardi Gras party. Typically, the traditional token is a tiny nonedible plastic baby. If you're not inclined to use a plastic baby (found in specialty baking supply stores), a whole shelled pecan works. Traditional Mardi Gras king cakes are usually decorated with unnaturally colored sugars. Although it is not as vibrant, I prefer to use the colored sugar that is naturally dyed. Naturally colored sugar can be found in most health-oriented grocery stores nationwide.

10 to 12 servings

1 package active dry yeast
1 teaspoon granulated sugar
¼ cup warm water
1 egg
1 cup sour cream
2 tablespoons canola oil
¼ cup granulated sugar
1 teaspoon salt
3 to 3½ cups unbleached all-purpose flour
4 ounces (block-style) ⅓ less fat cream cheese, at room temperature
3 tablespoons butter, melted
¼ cup granulated sugar
1 teaspoon cinnamon
½ cup pecans, chopped, plus 1 whole pecan for the prize
1½ cups confectioners' sugar
2 tablespoons milk
2 tablespoons butter, melted
¼ teaspoon vanilla
Naturally dyed yellow, green, and blue granulated colored sugar

1. Combine the yeast, sugar, and warm water in a large bowl. Stir until the yeast dissolves. Proof the yeast for 5 to 10 minutes.
2. Beat the egg in a medium bowl and then add the sour cream, oil, sugar, and salt. Whisk until well combined. Add the flour 1 cup at a time. When the dough begins to pull away from the sides of the bowl, turn out onto a floured board, and knead until smooth and elastic.
3. Transfer the dough to a floured surface and roll the dough into a 12-inch x 24-inch rectangle. If the dough resists, let it rest for a few minutes and then try again. Let the dough rest while you prepare the filling.
4. Combine the cream cheese, melted butter, sugar, and cinnamon in a small bowl, and mix until well blended. Spread the mixture evenly over the dough and top the mixture with pecans.
5. Lightly oil a rimmed baking sheet with cooking spray. Starting from the 24-inch part of the dough, begin rolling it into a long rope. Carefully transfer the rope to the baking sheet, and place it seam side down. Shape it into a ring, and pinch the ends together. Cover with a kitchen towel, and let it rest for 1 hour.
6. Preheat the oven to 375°F.
7. Bake the pastry for 25 to 28 minutes. Allow it to cool for about 10 minutes.
8. Cut a small slit anywhere in the bottom of the pastry cake, and insert the reserved pecan or token.
9. Combine the confectioners' sugar with the milk in a medium bowl, and then add the butter and vanilla, and whisk until fully combined. Spoon the glaze over the cooled cake. Sprinkle the colored sugars in alternating ribbons, 1 to 2 inches wide, over the top of the glaze.
10. To serve, slice cake into desired-sized slices.

CARDAMOM-INFUSED CRANBERRY COBBLER CAKE

I'm not a pumpkin pie enthusiast, so when thoughts of planning our Thanksgiving dinner come to mind, I go on a quest to invent something atypical, albeit seasonal, to serve for dessert. After my cookbook *Tasting the Seasons* was published, I tested a series of recipes for a popular dessert, strawberry cobbler cake. I changed the fruit according to the season and discovered that just about any fruit turned out a successful cobbler cake. Cranberries were no exception; the contrast of tart and sweet was very well received. The cardamom taste—best described as having a floral and ginger scent with a strong hint of citrus—is very pronounced. If you're not certain about the distinct flavor, cut back to 1 teaspoon. This cake is best served hot from the oven with coconut or vanilla ice cream.

8 servings

1 package (12 ounces) fresh cranberries, washed
1 cup unbleached all-purpose flour
1 cup granulated sugar
1½ teaspoons ground cardamom
1 teaspoon baking powder
¼ teaspoon salt
4 tablespoons butter, cut into chunks
¼ cup milk
1 tablespoon cornstarch
1 cup cold water

1. Preheat the oven to 350°F.
2. Place the cranberries in an 11 x 7 x 2-inch baking dish.
3. Combine the flour, sugar, ground cardamom, baking powder, and salt in a medium bowl. Drop the butter chunks into the flour mixture. Cut in the butter with two knives (making slicing motions), or use your fingertips to incorporate until the mixture is somewhat crumbly. Add the milk and stir until fully combined. Dollop the batter over the cranberries. (The batter is thick and more like dough than batter.) Don't worry if it doesn't cover the cranberries completely; the final water/cornstarch mixture and the baking process will evenly distribute the batter.

4. Combine the cornstarch with the water in a medium bowl. Stir until the cornstarch dissolves. Pour the mixture evenly over the batter, stirring as you pour, to keep the cornstarch evenly distributed with the water.

5. Bake the cobbler cake for 45 to 50 minutes or until lightly browned and bubbly. Serve hot from the oven with ice cream.

FRESH STRAWBERRY CAKE

When strawberries come into season, this simple and delectable cake makes its debut. It's delicious topped with dollops of whipped cream.

6 servings

3 cups strawberries, cut into bite-sized pieces
2 eggs
⅔ cup granulated sugar
1 teaspoon vanilla
½ cup (1 stick) butter, melted
1 cup unbleached all-purpose flour

1. Preheat the oven to 350°F.
2. Generously oil a 9-inch pie plate with cooking spray.
3. Arrange the strawberries in the bottom of the pie plate.
4. Beat the eggs in a large bowl on medium speed and gradually add the sugar. Add the vanilla and butter, and continue to beat until well combined. Slowly add the flour. Top the strawberries with the batter. (The batter doesn't have to cover the strawberries completely.)
5. Bake for 30 to 40 minutes or until light brown and bubbly. Serve immediately.

LEMON AND RICOTTA APPLE CAKE

This delicious cake is made incredibly moist by the apple and creamy ricotta. It turns a beautiful shade of chestnut brown, so don't think you've overbaked it. Just about any variety of apple works in this recipe; my preference is Gala. Apples tend to brown very quickly, so grate the apple just before adding it to the cake batter.

6 to 8 servings

½ cup (1 stick) butter, softened
1 tablespoon canola oil
1⅛ cups granulated sugar
2 eggs
1¼ cups unbleached all-purpose flour
1 tablespoon baking powder
¼ teaspoon salt
1 cup ricotta
2 teaspoons lemon zest
1 apple, peeled and grated (1 cup)
Confectioners' sugar for dusting the top of the cake

1. Preheat the oven to 400°F.
2. Generously butter a 9 x 1½-inch cake pan, and then dust the pan with flour.
3. Beat the butter and oil in a large bowl, and slowly add the sugar and beat on medium speed until light and fluffy. Lower the speed and add the eggs one at a time, beating well after each addition. Add the flour, baking powder, and salt, and beat until well blended. Add the ricotta, lemon zest, and grated apple, and incorporate until fully combined.
4. Transfer the batter to the prepared cake pan and bake for 30 to 40 minutes or until the cake is chestnut brown and a toothpick inserted in the center comes out clean.
5. Allow the cake to cool before transferring to a platter. Just before serving, dust the cake with confectioners' sugar.

APRICOT CHIA CAKE

This autumn-inspired cake recipe was invented when I was in the early stages of discussing the prospect of writing a cookbook about chia seeds. The assignment never came to fruition, but I had fun creating recipes using this trendy (at the time) seed. When chia seeds are added to liquid, they expand. Here they get soaked in buttermilk for 20 minutes, turning the mixture into a thickness much like sour cream. This recipe uses the recipe for autumn spice blend on page 148. If you're not inclined to prepare the blend, Spice Hunter Hot Buttered Rum Mix, available online, is a fine replacement.

6 to 8 servings

1 cup buttermilk
¼ cup chia seeds
½ cup canola oil
¾ cup granulated sugar
¼ cup autumn spice blend
2 eggs
1¼ cups unbleached all-purpose flour
1 tablespoon baking powder
¼ teaspoon salt
1 cup dried apricots, chopped
Confectioners' sugar for dusting the top of the cake

1. Preheat the oven to 400°F.
2. Generously oil a 9 x 1½-inch cake pan with cooking spray, and then dust the pan with flour.
3. Combine the buttermilk and chia seeds in a medium bowl. Allow the mixture to soak for 20 minutes.
4. Beat the canola oil in a large bowl on medium speed and slowly add the sugar and the autumn spice blend. Lower the speed and add the eggs one at a time, beating well after each addition. Add the flour, baking powder, and salt, and beat until well blended. Add the buttermilk/chia mixture and apricots, and incorporate until well distributed.
5. Transfer the batter to the prepared cake pan and bake for 35 minutes or until a toothpick inserted in the center of the cake comes out clean.
6. Allow the cake to cool before transferring to a serving platter. Just before serving, dust the top with confectioners' sugar.

CLOVE-SPIKED RED PLUM CAKE

When red plums are abundant at the farmers' market, I'm always anxious to make this beautiful cake. Plan accordingly; this is a yeast cake and needs to rise before it goes into the oven. McCutcheon's plum preserves is my favorite brand; see the Product Reference Guide, page 233.

8 servings

1¾ cups unbleached all-purpose flour
¼ cup granulated sugar
½ teaspoon salt
1 package active dry yeast
2 tablespoons butter, softened
½ cup hot water
1 egg
1½ cups fresh, ripe plums (about 2 medium), peeled and chopped
3 tablespoons granulated sugar
¼ teaspoon ground cloves
½ cup plum preserves

1. Combine ½ cup of flour, sugar, salt, and dry yeast in a large bowl. Add the butter and beat with an electric mixer for a few seconds on medium speed. Gradually add the hot water, and continue to beat for 2 minutes on medium speed while scraping the sides of the bowl. Add the egg and ½ cup of the flour. Switch to high speed and beat for 2 minutes, scraping the sides of the bowl. Stir in the remaining ¾ cup of flour and mix until well blended.

2. Lightly coat a 9 x 1½-inch cake pan with cooking spray. Spread the batter into the pan. (The batter will be thick and sticky, so don't be concerned if you can't spread it evenly. The rising process will evenly distribute the mixture.) Top the batter with the chopped plums.

3. Combine the sugar and cloves in a small bowl. Sprinkle the mixture over the plums.

4. Cover the cake with plastic wrap and allow the cake to rise in a warm, draft-free place for an hour or until double in bulk.

5. Preheat the oven to 400°F.

6. Bake the cake for 25 minutes. Allow it to cool for 10 minutes before carefully transferring it to a serving platter.

7. Heat the plum preserves in a small saucepan over low heat. Spoon the warm preserves evenly over the cake. Serve immediately.

STRAWBERRY-AND-CREAM-FILLED ROLLED CAKE

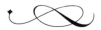

I offer my most enthusiastic "You-can-do-it" in the introduction to this chapter, because rolled cakes are a lot easier than you think. I teach rolled cake classes, and participants are amazed how easy it is. If you've never embarked on this culinary adventure, don't be daunted by the task. Not only is the outcome gratifying, it is impressive also. (And truly, it does not matter if the cake breaks when you roll it in the towel!) If there are cracks in the final roll, those imperfections make it look homemade—in an inviting way. Plan accordingly; the cake is best made a day in advance.

10 to 12 servings

1 cup unbleached all-purpose flour
½ teaspoon baking soda
½ teaspoon baking powder
¼ teaspoon salt
¾ cup granulated sugar
3 eggs
⅔ cup tapioca pudding
1 package (8 ounces, block-style) ⅓ less fat cream cheese, at room temperature
6 tablespoons butter, softened
1 cup confectioners' sugar
1 teaspoon vanilla
¼ cup strawberry preserves

1. Preheat the oven to 350°F.
2. Lightly oil a 12½ x 17½ x 1-inch rimmed baking sheet (jelly roll pan) with cooking spray and then line the pan with parchment paper, allowing enough paper to drape over all sides of the pan. Lightly coat the parchment paper with cooking spray and then lightly dust with flour. Set the prepared pan aside.
3. Combine the flour, baking soda, baking powder, salt, and sugar in a medium bowl.
4. Beat the eggs in a large bowl, add the pudding, and beat until well combined. Add the flour mixture and beat on medium speed until incorporated. Spread the batter evenly into the prepared baking sheet (it will seem like there's not enough batter, but there is), and bake for 10 minutes.
5. While the cake is baking, use a flour sifter to generously dust a kitchen cloth (the cloth should be a little larger than the size of the cake) with confectioners' sugar.

6. When the cake has baked, immediately remove the cake from the baking sheet (lifting up the two opposite corners of the parchment paper) and carefully flip the cake onto the prepared kitchen towel. Gently pull off the parchment paper.

7. Starting at the narrow end, roll the cake with the towel. Cool the cake wrapped in the towel on a wire rack for about 30 minutes.

8. While the cake is cooling, prepare the filling. Blend the cream cheese with the butter in a large bowl and beat until well combined. Add the confectioners' sugar and vanilla, and beat for about 2 minutes on medium speed. Add the strawberry preserves and beat until fully blended.

9. Carefully unroll the cake and spread the cream cheese filling evenly over the entire flat surface of the cake (while the cake is still on the towel). Gently re-roll the cake without the towel. (If some of the cake sticks to the towel, use your fingers or a flat metal spatula to ease it gently off the towel. Don't worry if the cake breaks as you're rolling it.) Cover the cake with plastic wrap (pull enough plastic wrap from the roll so that you have enough to tightly cover both ends of the roll) and refrigerate overnight.

10. Remove the cake from the refrigerator about 1 hour prior to serving.

11. To serve, cut the cake into 1-inch-thick slices.

CHOCOLATE-AND-CARAMEL-FILLED ROLLED CAKE

This cake is a crowd-pleaser! Plan accordingly; the cake is best made a day in advance.

10 to 12 servings

¾ cup unbleached all-purpose flour
½ teaspoon baking soda
½ teaspoon baking powder
¼ teaspoon salt
¼ cup cocoa powder
¾ cup granulated sugar
3 eggs
⅔ cup chocolate pudding
1 package (8 ounces, block-style) ⅓ less fat cream cheese, at room temperature
½ cup cream caramel sauce

1. Preheat the oven to 350°F.
2. Lightly oil a 12½ x 17½ x 1-inch rimmed baking sheet (jelly roll pan) with cooking spray, and then line the pan with parchment paper, allowing enough paper to drape over all sides of the pan. Lightly coat the parchment paper with cooking spray and then lightly dust with flour. A flour sifter works great. Set the prepared pan aside.
3. Combine the flour, baking soda, baking powder, salt, cocoa powder, and sugar in a medium bowl.
4. Beat the eggs in a large bowl with an electric mixer. Add the chocolate pudding and beat until well combined. Add the flour mixture and beat on medium speed until incorporated. Spread the batter evenly in the pan (it will seem like there's not enough batter, but there is), and bake for 10 minutes.
5. While the cake is baking, use a flour sifter to dust a kitchen cloth with a generous amount of confectioners' sugar. The cloth should be a little larger than the size of the cake.
6. As soon as the cake has baked, lift up the two opposite corners of the parchment paper to remove it from the baking pan, and then carefully flip the cake onto the prepared kitchen towel. Gently pull off the parchment paper.

7. Starting at the narrow end, roll the cake with the towel. Cool the cake wrapped in the towel on a wire rack for about 30 minutes.

8. While the cake is cooling, prepare the filling. Combine the cream cheese with the caramel sauce in a medium bowl and whisk until fully blended.

9. While the cake is still on the towel, carefully unroll it. Spread the cream cheese filling evenly over the entire flat surface of the cake. Gently re-roll the cake without the towel. (If some of the cake sticks to the towel, use your fingers or a flat metal spatula to ease it gently off the towel. Don't worry if the cake breaks as you're rolling it.) Cover the cake with plastic wrap (pull enough plastic wrap from the roll so that you have enough to cover both ends of the roll) and refrigerate overnight.

10. Remove the cake from the refrigerator about 1 hour prior to serving.

11. To serve, cut the cake into 1-inch-thick slices.

PEACHES-AND-CREAM-FILLED ROLLED CAKE

Is there anything more complementary than peaches and cream? Plan accordingly; this cake is best made a day in advance.

10 to 12 servings

¾ cup unbleached all-purpose flour
½ teaspoon baking soda
½ teaspoon baking powder
¼ teaspoon salt
½ cup granulated sugar
3 eggs
⅔ cup tapioca pudding
1 package (8 ounces, block-style) ⅓ less fat cream cheese, at room temperature
½ cup peach marmalade
1 teaspoon vanilla

1. Preheat the oven to 350°F.
2. Lightly oil a 12½ x 17½ x 1-inch rimmed baking sheet (jelly roll pan) with cooking spray and then line the pan with parchment paper, allowing enough paper to drape over all sides of the pan. Lightly coat the parchment paper with cooking spray and then lightly dust with flour. Set the prepared pan aside.
3. Combine the flour, baking soda, baking powder, salt, and sugar in a medium bowl.
4. Beat the eggs in a large bowl, and then add the tapioca pudding and beat until well combined. Add the flour mixture and beat on medium speed until incorporated. Spread the batter evenly into the prepared baking sheet (it will seem like there's not enough batter, but there is), and bake the cake for 10 minutes.
5. While the cake is baking, use a flour sifter to generously dust a kitchen cloth (the cloth should be a little larger than the size of the cake) with confectioners' sugar.
6. As soon as the cake has baked, lift up the two opposite corners of the parchment paper to remove the cake from the baking sheet and carefully flip the cake onto the prepared kitchen towel. Gently pull off the parchment paper.
7. Starting at the narrow end, roll the cake with the towel. Cool the cake wrapped in a towel on a wire rack for about 30 minutes.

8. While the cake is cooling, prepare the filling. Beat the cream cheese in a medium bowl, and then add the vanilla and the peach marmalade. Beat for about 2 minutes on medium speed.

9. While the cake is still on the towel, carefully unroll it. Spread the cream cheese filling evenly over the entire flat surface. Gently re-roll the cake without the towel. (If some of the cake sticks to the towel, use your fingers or a flat metal spatula to ease it gently off the towel. Don't worry if the cake breaks as you're rolling it.) Cover the cake with plastic wrap (pull enough plastic wrap from the roll so that you have enough to cover both ends of the roll) and refrigerate overnight.

10. Remove the cake from the refrigerator about 1 hour prior to serving.

11. To serve, cut the cake into 1-inch-thick slices.

CHOCOLATE-COCONUT-AND-GINGERED-CRANBERRY-CREAM-FILLED ROLLED CAKE

The combination for this moist, cream-filled cake came into being because of some leftover gingered cranberry sauce (see page 150). If you're not inclined to make that cranberry recipe, use your favorite cranberry sauce. Plan accordingly; the cake is best made a day in advance.

10 to 12 servings

¾ cup unbleached all-purpose flour
½ teaspoon baking soda
½ teaspoon baking powder
¼ teaspoon salt
¼ cup cocoa powder
¾ cup granulated sugar
3 eggs
⅔ cup chocolate pudding
1 package (8 ounces, block-style) ⅓ less fat cream cheese, at room temperature
¾ cup gingered cranberry sauce
½ cup shredded sweetened coconut
½ cup confectioners' sugar
1 teaspoon vanilla
Confectioners' sugar, for dusting finished cake

1. Preheat the oven to 350°F.
2. Lightly oil a 12½ x 17½ x 1-inch rimmed baking sheet (jelly roll pan) with cooking spray and then line the pan with parchment paper, allowing enough paper to drape over all sides of the pan. Lightly coat the parchment paper with cooking spray and then lightly dust with flour. Set the prepared pan aside.
3. Combine the flour, baking soda, baking powder, salt, cocoa powder, and sugar in a medium bowl.

4. Beat the eggs in a large bowl, and then add the chocolate pudding and beat until well blended. Add the flour mixture and beat on medium speed until incorporated. Spread the batter evenly onto the prepared baking sheet (it will seem like there's not enough batter, but there is), and bake for 10 minutes.

5. While the cake is baking, use a flour sifter to generously dust a kitchen towel (the towel should be larger than the size of the cake) with confectioners' sugar.

6. As soon as the cake has baked, lift up the two opposite corners of the parchment paper to remove the cake from the baking sheet and carefully flip the cake onto the prepared kitchen towel. Gently pull off the parchment paper.

7. Starting at the narrow end, roll the cake with the towel. Cool the cake wrapped in the towel on a wire rack for about 30 minutes.

8. While the cake is cooling, prepare the filling. Beat the cream cheese with the cranberry sauce in a large bowl until well combined. Add the coconut, confectioners' sugar, and vanilla, and beat for about 2 minutes on medium speed.

9. While the cake is still on the towel, carefully unroll it and spread the cranberry filling evenly over the entire flat surface of the cake. Gently re-roll the cake without the towel. (If some of the cake sticks to the towel, use your fingers or a flat spatula to ease it gently off the towel. Don't worry if the cake breaks as you're rolling it.) Cover the cake with plastic wrap (pull enough plastic wrap from the roll so that you have enough to cover both ends of the roll) and refrigerate overnight.

10. Remove the cake from the refrigerator about 1 hour prior to serving.

11. To serve, cut the cake into 1-inch-thick slices.

CARAMEL CHOCOLATE PIE WITH SALTY PRETZEL CRUST

After we sampled the first bite, we were hooked. But just to make sure, I shared some samples with a group of taste-testers. The look in their eyes revealed a lot and pretty much summed up our reaction: sweet and salty, and a fabulous dessert to serve anyone who adores chocolate and caramel. The unwavering conclusion is that this decadent dessert is an absolute winner. Plan accordingly; the interior of this dessert cooks for about 2 hours, and then once it has cooled, it needs to be refrigerated for several hours. If you want to serve it the day you plan to make it, start first thing in the morning.

8 to 10 servings

12 pretzel rods, about 1¼ cups
1 stick (½ cup) butter, melted
¼ cup brown sugar
2 cans (14 ounces each) sweetened condensed milk
½ cup heavy whipping cream
4 ounces bittersweet chocolate, broken into chunks

1. Preheat the oven to 350°F.
2. Process the pretzel rods in a food processor until crushed. Add the melted butter and brown sugar, and pulse until the mixture is well combined. Transfer the mixture (reserve ¼ cup for the top of the pie) to a 9-inch pie plate and press the mixture into the bottom and sides of the pie plate. Bake for 10 minutes.
3. Reset the oven temperature to 425°F.
4. Add enough hot water to fill a 13 x 9 x 2-inch baking dish one-third full. Transfer the condensed milk to an 11 x 7 x 2-inch baking dish and cover the dish with tinfoil. Place the 11 x 7 x 2-inch baking dish into a 13 x 9 x 2-inch baking dish. Carefully place the baking dishes in the oven and cook for 2 hours or until the mixture is thick and caramel colored. Stir the mixture every 30 minutes and add more water to the 13 x 9 x 2-inch baking dish if needed. (Be careful not to get a steam burn when removing the tinfoil to stir the mixture.) As the mixture thickens, it begins to get lumpy. Don't worry; the lumps sort out during the chilling process.
5. Spread the caramel evenly over the salty pretzel crust. Allow the mixture to cool for about a half hour, then refrigerate for at least 4 hours.
6. Bring the cream to a gentle boil in a small pan over moderate heat. Remove from heat and add the chocolate. Stir until smooth.

7. Allow the chocolate mixture to cool for about 45 minutes.
8. Pour the chocolate evenly over the caramel mixture. Sprinkle the reserved salty pretzel mixture over the chocolate. Cover and refrigerate for several hours before serving.

CARAMEL CREAM PIE WITH SALTY PRETZEL CRUST

This is very similar to the caramel chocolate pie with salty pretzel crust recipe on page 214. Here I've omitted the chocolate and added sweet whipped cream as the topping for the caramel. I prepared it for a dinner party, and the consensus was an emphatic "Winner!" Plan accordingly; the interior of this dessert cooks for about 2 hours, and once cool, it gets refrigerated for several hours. If you want to serve it the day you plan to make it, start first thing in the morning.

8 to 10 servings

12 pretzel rods, about 1¼ cups
1 stick (½ cup) butter, melted
¼ cup brown sugar
2 cans (14 ounces each) sweetened condensed milk
2 cups heavy whipping cream
2 tablespoons confectioners' sugar

1. Place either the mixing bowl or beaters in the freezer. (One or the other needs to be very cold for the cream to properly whip.)
2. Preheat the oven to 350°F.
3. Process the pretzel rods in a food processor and pulse until they are crushed. Add the melted butter and brown sugar, and pulse the mixture until combined. Set aside ¼ cup of the pretzel mixture for the topping. Transfer the remaining mixture to a 9-inch pie plate. Bake for about 10 minutes. Set aside.
4. Reset the oven temperature to 425°F.
5. Add enough hot water to fill a 13 x 9 x 2-inch baking dish one-third full. Transfer the condensed milk to an 11 x 7 x 2-inch baking dish, and cover the dish with tinfoil. Place the 11 x 7 x 2-inch baking dish into the 13 x 9 x 2-inch baking dish. Carefully place the baking dishes in the oven and cook for about 2 hours, until the mixture is thick and caramel colored. Stir the mixture every 30 minutes and add more water to the 13 x 9 x 2-inch baking dish if needed. (Be careful not to get a steam burn when removing the tinfoil to stir the mixture.) As the mixture thickens, it begins to get lumpy. Don't worry; the lumps sort out during the chilling process.
6. Spread the caramel evenly over the salty pretzel crust. Allow the mixture to cool for about a half hour, then refrigerate for at least 4 hours.

7. After the pie has refrigerated, pour the whipping cream into a medium bowl and beat on medium speed. Add the confectioners' sugar. When the cream thickens, increase the speed and continue to beat until stiff peaks form. (Be careful not to overbeat or the cream will turn to butter.) Top the caramel pie with the whipped cream and sprinkle the reserved salty pretzel mixture on top. Serve immediately.

CHOCOLATE, COCONUT, AND PEANUT BUTTER PIE

Fair warning: This is a rich-tasting, melt-in-your-mouth, ultra-sweet dessert. Because it's so rich, I cut the wedges smaller than the typical pie wedge. Plan accordingly; the pie cools for 1 hour and then needs to be refrigerated for about 4 hours.

12 servings

½ cup (1 stick) butter
1½ cups graham crackers (about 10 crackers)
7 ounces shredded sweetened coconut
1 can (14 ounces) sweetened condensed milk
1 package (12 ounces) semisweet chocolate chips
½ cup chunky natural peanut butter

1. Preheat the oven to 325°F.
2. Place the butter in the pie plate and allow the butter to melt in the oven.
3. Process the graham crackers in a food processor until they are crushed.
4. When the butter has melted, sprinkle the graham cracker crumbs evenly over the butter. Top the buttered graham cracker crumbs with the shredded coconut, distributing the coconut evenly over the graham crackers. Pour the sweetened condensed milk over the coconut, making certain to get all the condensed milk out of the can.
5. Bake for 25 minutes or until lightly browned.
6. Melt the chocolate chips with the peanut butter in a small pan over moderate heat. Stir to combine well. Spread the chocolate/peanut butter mixture evenly over the coconut/condensed milk mixture. Cool for 1 hour. Cover and refrigerate for about 4 hours.
7. Remove from refrigerator about 15 minutes before cutting into wedges.

COCONUT CUSTARD PIE

This creamy, crustless pie is super-simple to assemble. It got rave reviews from taste-testers who described it as having a pudding-like, custardy texture—the perfect contrast with the shredded coconut that inexplicably turns into a crispy crust! My friend Katherine, who loves to eat chocolate and coconut together, loves this pie topped with chocolate sauce. I prefer the coconut flavor without the addition of chocolate. Coconut milk naturally separates and hardens—it will become fluid when heated. Shake the can well before opening and stir until fully blended before adding to the remaining ingredients.

8 servings

4 tablespoons butter
1 cup granulated sugar
2 eggs
½ cup unbleached all-purpose flour
¾ teaspoon baking powder
¼ teaspoon salt
1 can (14 ounces) coconut milk
2 cups sweetened shredded coconut
Chocolate sauce (optional)

1. Preheat the oven to 350°F.
2. Lightly oil a 9-inch pie plate with cooking spray.
3. Melt the butter in a small saucepan over low heat. Transfer the butter to a large bowl.
4. Whisk the melted butter with the sugar. Add the eggs and whisk until smooth. Add the flour, baking powder, and salt. Whisk until well combined. Stir in the coconut milk and shredded coconut, and then mix well.
5. Transfer the mixture to the pie plate and bake for 55 to 60 minutes or until golden brown and firm to the touch. Allow the pie to cool completely before serving. Pass the chocolate sauce (if desired) to your guests.

RHUBARB PIE

I found this recipe buried among my mother's vast collection. It was scribbled by hand and came without details. I have an affection for rhubarb, and I'm always excited when I discover this unappreciated and lesser-known early spring vegetable in a recipe. The first time I prepared the pie, I thought the recipe was in error because the mixture that goes on top of the rhubarb is very thick. I placed it in the oven, closed the door, and thought, "I don't think this is going to be a very good pie." But I was mistaken. We ate the whole pie in one sitting—just the two of us! If you prefer a non-hydrogenated vegetable shortening, see the Product Reference Guide, page 233, for my suggestion. Measure and refrigerate the flour for about an hour prior to making the crust.

6 to 8 servings

1½ cups unbleached all-purpose flour, cold
½ teaspoon salt
¼ cup shortening
½ cup cold water
4 cups rhubarb, sliced about ½-inch thick
1½ cups granulated sugar
3 egg yolks
½ cup unbleached all-purpose flour
2 tablespoons milk
A pinch of nutmeg

1. Combine 1½ cups of flour and salt in a large bowl. Add the shortening to the flour mixture. Use your fingers to mesh the flour with the shortening, and mix until the mixture is coarse. Slowly add the cold water. (Add more water if necessary to make a soft dough.) Using your hands, bring the flour mixture together until the ingredients are fully incorporated.
2. Lightly flour a work surface. Take two-thirds of the dough and roll it into a 12-inch circle. Transfer the dough to a 9-inch pie plate and flute the edges using the dough that overlaps the pie plate. Prick the shell with a fork in several places to ensure even baking. Set aside the remaining dough and cover until ready to use.
3. Preheat the oven to 400°F.
4. Place the rhubarb in the unbaked pie shell.
5. Combine the sugar, egg yolks, ½ cup of flour, milk, and nutmeg in a medium bowl, and blend until incorporated. Spoon the mixture over the rhubarb. (The mixture is very thick and doesn't have to be spread perfectly; it will sort out while baking.)

6. Roll the remaining dough into a 9-inch round. Place on top of the mixture. Seal the edges of the bottom crust with the top crust. Using a sharp knife, make a few incisions on the top of the pie crust. (To avoid any possible spillage on the oven floor, place the pie on a rimmed baking sheet.)
7. Bake for 20 minutes at 400°F. Reduce the oven temperature to 350°F and bake for an additional 30 to 40 minutes or until light brown and bubbly. Allow the pie to cool before cutting.

BITTERSWEET CHOCOLATE COOKIES WITH SEA SALT

If the combination of bittersweet chocolate and sea salt is all you need to satisfy your chocolate craving, then this cookie is the one for you. Plan accordingly, especially if your craving is irrepressible; the dough has to refrigerate overnight.

3½ dozen cookies

½ cup granulated sugar
½ cup light brown sugar
10 tablespoons butter
1 egg
1 teaspoon vanilla
1 cup unbleached all-purpose flour
¾ teaspoon baking powder
¾ teaspoon baking soda
¾ teaspoon salt
8 ounces bittersweet chocolate, cut into chip-sized pieces
Coarse sea salt

1. Combine the granulated sugar with the brown sugar in a large bowl.
2. Melt the butter in a medium saucepan over moderate heat. Cook the butter until chestnut brown, stirring frequently—this will take several minutes. (There is a narrow window between brown butter and burnt butter, so watch closely.) Pour the hot brown butter over the sugar; don't stir. Refrigerate the mixture for about 45 minutes.
3. After 45 minutes, beat the brown butter/sugar mixture on medium speed until light and somewhat fluffy. Add the egg and beat until fully combined. Add the vanilla and beat until incorporated.
4. Combine the flour with the baking powder, baking soda, and salt in a medium bowl. Add the flour mixture to the brown butter/sugar mixture and mix until combined. Stir in the chocolate pieces. Cover the mixture and refrigerate overnight.
5. Allow the dough to come to room temperature for about 1 hour or until it's pliable.
6. Preheat the oven to 350°F.
7. Line 2 rimmed baking sheets with parchment paper.

8. Form the dough into balls, about 1 inch in diameter. Arrange the balls on the baking sheet about 2 inches apart, or 12 per baking sheet. Flatten each ball slightly with the palm of your hand. Sprinkle each cookie with coarse sea salt.

9. Bake for 14 minutes, switching baking trays halfway through the baking time.

10. Allow the cookies to stand on the baking sheet for about 5 minutes before transferring to a wire rack to cool.

CHOCOLATE FUDGE AND PISTACHIO NUT COOKIES

Just about every person my mother played bridge with was a fantastic cook. I found this cookie recipe among her immense collection. At the top of the barely legible recipe—heavy with food stains—were four stars, my mother's coding for what she thought was an excellent, go-to recipe. I added pistachios (the original recipe called for walnuts or pecans) and sea salt with great flavor results.

5 dozen cookies

¼ cup (½ stick) butter
12 ounces semisweet chocolate chips
1 can (14 ounces) sweetened condensed milk
1 teaspoon vanilla
1 cup unbleached all-purpose flour
1 cup chopped pistachio nuts
Sea salt

1. Preheat the oven to 350°F.
2. Lightly oil a baking sheet with cooking spray.
3. Melt the butter, chocolate chips, and sweetened condensed milk in a medium pan over moderate heat. As the ingredients begin to melt, stir to combine. Heat until melted and well blended.
4. Remove the pan from the heat, add the vanilla, and stir until fully incorporated. Add the flour ½ cup at a time, stirring well after each addition. Stir in the pistachio nuts.
5. Measure about 1 tablespoon of cookie dough for each cookie and place on the prepared baking sheet about 2 inches apart, or 12 per baking sheet.
6. Bake for 7 to 8 minutes. Allow the cookies to cool for about 1 minute before transferring to a wire rack. Sprinkle with sea salt.

LEMON CRINKLE COOKIES

If you're a fan of lemon, these are sure to please.

About 5 dozen cookies

½ cup butter, softened
1 cup granulated sugar
½ teaspoons vanilla
1 egg
Lemon zest from 1 whole lemon
1 tablespoon fresh lemon juice
¼ teaspoon salt
¼ teaspoon baking powder
¼ teaspoon baking soda
1½ cups unbleached all-purpose flour
½ cup powdered sugar

1. Preheat the oven to 350°F.
2. Line 2 baking sheets with parchment paper.
3. Cream the butter with the sugar in a large bowl. Add the vanilla, egg, lemon zest, and juice. Beat until light and fluffy. Add the salt, baking powder, baking soda, and flour. Mix until fully combined.
4. Place the powdered sugar in a medium bowl.
5. Roll a heaping teaspoon of dough into a ball and roll in the powdered sugar. Repeat with the remaining dough and place the balls on the prepared baking sheets, 12 cookies per sheet.
6. Bake for 10 to 12 minutes (switch baking sheets halfway through cooking time to ensure even baking) or until the bottoms of the cookies are barely brown.
7. Transfer the cookies to a wire rack to cool completely.

ALMOND LACE COOKIES

I came across this recipe when I was rummaging through my mother's recipe collection. It stood out among a pile of dessert recipes because she had marked the recipe with four stars—her code for excellent. The recipe was written using a green felt-tip pen, and I could barely decipher some of the ingredients' measurements because the ink had bled. The measurements were questionable, and they would make even a seasoned cook's eyebrows go aflutter. The recipe called for 1¼ teaspoons of flour. Given this small amount, I wondered what would keep these predominantly butter-and nut-filled cookies from not spreading all over the baking pan. Logically, it seemed like they would need more flour to hold the ingredients together. After some contemplation, I decided not to add more flour. I placed tiny amounts far apart on the cookie sheet, took a deep breath, and placed them in the oven. They came out so thin we could see through them. These crispy, nutty, buttery lace cookies lived up to my mother's four-star rating. They are delectable, paper thin and very fragile. Following the directions precisely is the key to the success of these cookies.

About 3½ dozen cookies

¼ cup (½ stick) butter
⅓ cup almonds, ground
¼ cup granulated sugar
1¼ teaspoons flour
A pinch of salt
1 tablespoon milk

1. Preheat the oven to 350°F.
2. Coat 2 rimmed baking sheets with cooking spray and then dust them with flour.
3. Melt the butter in a small pan over moderately low heat. Add the ground almonds, sugar, flour, and salt. Cook, stirring occasionally, until the sugar has dissolved. Add the milk and stir until combined. Let the mixture stand for about 5 minutes.
4. Measure and place ½ teaspoon of the mixture onto the prepared baking sheets. Be exact in your measurement because any more and the cookies will run into each other. You should have 8 cookies per sheet.
5. Bake for 6 to 7 minutes or until chestnut colored (check after 5 minutes). Switch baking pans halfway through the baking time.
6. Allow the cookies to cool on the baking sheet for 2 minutes (no longer), and then quickly and carefully transfer them to a wire rack to cool completely.

ALMOND COOKIES

If you're a fan of almonds, you will love these cookies. They are super-simple to assemble, using just three ingredients.

20 cookies

1 can (8 ounces) almond paste
½ cup granulated sugar
1 egg white

1. Place the oven rack in the center of the oven.
2. Preheat the oven to 325°F.
3. Line 2 rimmed baking sheets with parchment paper.
4. Break the almond paste into about 6 pieces and place in a food processor. Add the sugar and pulse until the sugar is combined with the almond paste—the mixture will look like coarse salt. Add the egg white and pulse until the mixture turns moist and sticky looking.
5. Measure 1 tablespoon for each cookie and roll it into a ball. (The mixture is super-sticky. If you lightly dampen your hands with water or oil before rolling the mixture into a ball, it will be easier to handle.) Flatten the cookies slightly with the palm of your hand and place them on the prepared baking sheet, 10 per sheet.
6. Bake for 20 minutes. Transfer the oven rack to the upper part of the oven and bake for an additional 6 to 8 minutes.
7. Transfer the cookies to a wire rack to cool.

FROZEN MARGARITA MARTINIS WITH SALTY PRETZEL CRUST

Instead of imbibing a predinner margarita, here is a fantastic-tasting warm-weather cocktail dessert. Fresh whipped cream and sweetened condensed milk are the smooth and creamy basis. Standard margarita ingredients—triple sec, tequila, and fresh lime juice—are added to give it that authentic margarita flavor. Sweet and buttery crushed pretzels top this divine and velvety-textured dessert— the perfect ending to a summer meal. It's simple to assemble, and I love that most of it can be prepared in advance—more time outside with family and friends. Take note; the mixture has to freeze for 3 to 4 hours before serving. Remember to place either the mixing bowl or beaters in the freezer for a few hours prior to whipping the cream.

6 servings

1½ cups pretzels (about 15 rods)
¼ cup granulated sugar
1 stick (½ cup) butter, melted
1 can (14 ounces) sweetened condensed milk
⅓ cup fresh lime juice
2 tablespoons triple sec
2 tablespoons tequila
2 teaspoons grated lime zest
8 ounces heavy whipping cream
Six slices of lime (garnish)

1. Process the pretzels in a food processor until crushed. Transfer to a medium bowl and combine the crushed pretzels with the sugar. Add the melted butter and stir until the ingredients are fully incorporated. Cover and set aside.
2. Whisk the sweetened condensed milk with the lime juice, triple sec, tequila, and lime zest in a large bowl. Set aside.
3. Pour the whipping cream into a medium bowl and beat on medium speed. When the cream thickens, increase the speed and continue to beat until stiff peaks form. (Be careful not to overbeat or the cream will turn to butter.) Fold the whipped cream into the sweetened condensed milk mixture. Transfer the mixture to a container with a tight-fitting lid and freeze for 3 to 4 hours or until firm.

4. Just prior to serving, divide the frozen mixture among six martini glasses. Garnish each glass with lime slices. Top each with the buttery pretzel mixture. Serve immediately.

COCONUT AND ROASTED PEANUT ICE CREAM WITH THAI BASIL

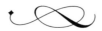

My friend Lena and I get together regularly and spend the day cooking. When my garden was brimming with Thai basil, Lena and I put it to work. We made homemade ice cream, adding Thai basil, coconut butter, and peanuts, and were thrilled with our endeavor. The ice cream should be soft enough so that you can easily fold in the ingredients. But if you let it get too soft, the peanuts will sink to the bottom.

4 servings

1 pint vanilla ice cream, semisoft
1 cup Thai basil leaves, roughly chopped (plus extra leaves for garnish)
½ cup peanuts, roasted, salted, and roughly chopped
2 tablespoons coconut butter

1. In a large bowl, combine the ice cream with the basil, peanuts, and coconut butter. Place the mixture in a container to accommodate and freeze until serving time.

CREAMY STRAWBERRY SOUP WITH AMARETTO

This ridiculously simple dessert soup is perfect to serve when strawberries are at the height of their season and locally plentiful. I don't recommend preparing it any other time of the year. Light and refreshing, it's a memorable end to any summer meal. For a glorious presentation, serve in chilled martini glasses. Plan accordingly; the soup needs to be refrigerated for several hours.

8 ½-cup servings

1 quart (5 cups) strawberries, capped, plus extra for garnishing glasses
8 ounces sour cream
¼ cup almond liqueur (aka Amaretto)
2 tablespoons brown sugar
¼ teaspoon almond extract
Garden-fresh mint leaves (garnish)

1. Place the martini glasses or soup bowls in the refrigerator to chill.
2. Combine the strawberries, sour cream, almond liqueur, brown sugar, and almond extract in a blender or food processor, and purée until silky smooth.
3. Transfer to a container, cover, and refrigerate for several hours or overnight.
4. Ladle the soup into the chilled martini glasses or soup bowls, garnish the rims with a strawberry, and float a pair of fresh mint leaves on the top of each serving. Serve immediately.

PRODUCT REFERENCE GUIDE

I'm often asked, "What size eggs do you use? Do you prefer salted or unsalted butter? What is neutral oil?" So, I've created a list that references those questions, as well as certain foods, products, and brands from the foremost companies I endorse that are used throughout the cookbook. These items are generally available in grocery stores nationwide, some universally. Several culinary tips are also included to help guide you.

ASPARAGUS: Choose thin, medium, or thick asparagus spears—it's really a matter of preference. I prefer medium-sized spears. To prepare, take each spear by its end and gently bend it in half. The spears will snap at approximately the point where tenderness begins. Asparagus is best consumed the day you purchase it.

BAKING POWDER: I prefer aluminum-free baking powder. Baking powder with aluminum tends to have a bitter "tinny" flavor. Most grocery stores nationwide carry aluminum-free baking powder.

BUTTER: Salted butter is used in the recipes in this cookbook.

BUTTERMILK: My mother used buttermilk repeatedly. I use it as frequently as she did, and it is called for in numerous recipes in all my cookbooks. Many people labor under the misconception that buttermilk is basically a buttery, high-fat milk. This couldn't be farther from the truth. Not only is there no butter, per se, in buttermilk, but it's actually lower in fat than milk. The "butter" in buttermilk is not an allusion to its butteriness, but rather an explanation of where this versatile fermented beverage comes from.

CHEESES: Freshly grated cheese is used in all the recipes, rather than cheese that was bought pre-grated. Any food that has been taken from its whole and grated or sliced loses its authentic flavor over time.

CHEESE, FETA: I'm partial to the flavor of Valbresso's feta, the brand used in all the recipes that call for feta in this cookbook. Feta does not have a rind or outer hard layer and is usually pressed into square or rectangular blocks. It dries out and sours quickly when removed from its brine. For that reason, blocks of packaged feta cheese are covered with brine and should be stored and kept refrigerated in the brine until used.

CHICKEN BROTH: The most flavorful and authentic store-bought I've taste-tested is Imagine organic chicken broth.

COCONUT MILK: I've tested many coconut milk brands, and Thai is my favorite for its authentic, rich coconut flavor. Coconut milk naturally separates and hardens—it will become fluid when heated. Shake the can well before opening and stir until fully blended before using, especially when adding to a recipe that won't be puréed or blended, as in many of the recipes for soup in this cookbook.

COCONUT, SHREDDED: Unless otherwise specified, shredded sweetened coconut is used.

COOKING OILS: Many oils line grocery store shelves, but not all oils are created equal in flavor, usage, or production. When buying vegetable oil, I highly recommend purchasing expeller-pressed organic oils because GMOs and hexane (a chemical) extraction are prohibited in nearly all organic oil production. To be sure, always check the label. Cold-pressed oils are of a higher quality because the lower processing temperatures preserve the flavor and characteristics of the oil. Refined oils are generally mild and devoid of flavor. Unrefined oils are less processed, have more flavor, and are often of a higher quality.

Because of its health-promoting properties, I like to use coconut oil whenever a neutral oil can be used. A good example is when I cook pancakes; it will add a mild hint of coconut flavor without altering the taste too much. I also use coconut oil whenever there is coconut in a recipe. It is best (unless you use a certain oil every day) to store oil in the refrigerator.

Certain oils are better for different types of cooking.

Baking: Canola (expeller-pressed), coconut, high-oleic safflower, palm, and sunflower oil work well.

Frying: Because they stand up well to heat, avocado, palm, peanut, sesame (not toasted), and sunflower oil are suitable.

Marinades and salad dressings: Canola (expeller-pressed), olive, peanut, toasted sesame, or walnut oil.

Sautéing: Many oils are great for sautéing—avocado, canola (expeller-pressed), coconut, grapeseed, high-oleic safflower, olive, sesame (not toasted), and sunflower oils.

Neutral (aka flavorless) oil: For oil that won't contribute to or alter the flavor of your dish—expeller-pressed canola, high-oleic safflower, and sunflower oil.

CREAM CHEESE: ⅓ less fat cream cheese (aka Neufchâtel cream cheese, or light cream cheese), block-style, is used in all the recipes that call for cream cheese. It has better blending qualities than full-fat cream cheese. Full-fat cream cheese can be used with the same results.

EGGS: Unless otherwise noted, large eggs are used in the recipes in this cookbook.

FLAXSEED: When a recipe calls for ground flaxseeds, a coffee grinder works perfectly to grind the seeds.

HORSERADISH: My favorite brand is Kelchner's prepared horseradish; it's the best I've tasted. It can be found in the refrigerated section (usually near the seafood or in the refrigerated grocery section) of most grocery stores nationwide.

JAMS, JELLIES, AND PRESERVES: When I don't traditionally preserve or I can't source a local vendor that does, I source Bonne Maman, McCutcheon's (love their plum preserves), and Stonewall Kitchen for their flavor and quality. Ginger preserves and pineapple preserves are not as common as some of the more familiar jams, jellies, and preserves. For ginger preserves, my favorite brands are from Dundee or Wilkin & Sons; they both have a pronounced ginger flavor. They can be found in upscale grocery stores or online. For pineapple, the best I've tasted is from Dillman Farm, available online.

MANGO, VARIETY: I am partial to the sweet, rich flavor of the Alphonso mango variety. It is one of the most popular varieties because of its intense sweetness and rich flavor. The Alphonso mango season typically begins in late April and runs until the beginning of September.

MILK: When milk is called for in a recipe, I use organic whole cow's milk, unless otherwise noted.

MUSHROOMS: Whether you get mushrooms from a mushroom farmer, from self-serving bins at the grocery store, or prepackaged, the size and weight of mushrooms varies. When you set out to prepare any of the recipes in this book that call for mushrooms and you have an uncertain amount you bought from the mushroom farmer or you can only find a 12-ounce package versus a 10-ounce package, wing it—can there ever be too many mushrooms? I feel confident your estimation for usage and choice (if you want to use a variation) will turn out a fine-tasting dish.

Unless otherwise noted, I use white mushrooms in the recipes. Their availability and versatility make them indispensable, and even though they lack some of the earthy intensity of their quirky-looking cousins, not everyone has access to the wide variety of mushrooms available.

MUSHROOM, SOUP: My preferred brand is Amy's cream of mushroom soup because it is chock-full of mushroom flavor.

PARSLEY: Fresh parsley is often called for in the cookbook, and sometimes in large quantities. One cup of loosely packed parsley will yield about ½ cup of minced parsley. To store a fresh bunch of parsley, wash, shake out any excess water, and snip the ends from the bunch. Fill a tall glass half full of water. Place the stems in the water and allow the parsley leaves to dry before covering with a plastic bag. The parsley will keep refrigerated for several days.

ROASTED VEGETABLES, HOW TO: I love to make big batches of roasted vegetables. I repurpose them throughout the week. I add them to sandwiches, spoon them over hummus, or toss them with cooked pasta. They also make a great topping for vegetarian or beef burgers and are delicious served with grilled beef. They are simple to prepare: Cut tomatoes and onions into quarters, slice carrots about ¼-inch thick, and cut bell peppers into chunks. Place the vegetables on a rimmed baking sheet, toss with olive oil, and sprinkle them with coarse salt. Roast them in a 400°F oven for 1 to 1½ hours (stirring every ½ hour) or until tender and slightly blackened.

SPAGHETTI SQUASH, HOW TO BAKE: Preheat the oven to 350°F. Cut the squash in half and remove the seeds. Place the squash halves cut side down in a baking dish that accommodates both halves. Add 1 to 2 inches of water to the baking dish—the halves should be partially submersed in the water. Bake uncovered for 30 to 45 minutes or until a fork goes easily through the thickest part of the squash halves. Remove the halves from the water bath and transfer to a platter. When the squash is cool enough to handle, use a fork to "rake" the strands from the halves.

SALT: So many of the salts on the market today have been heat processed and stripped of their natural trace minerals. I use Real Salt sea salt because it's unrefined and full of natural minerals and flavor—I'm convinced this makes a difference.

SEASONING SALTS: A.A. Borsari has a few seasoned salts that are used frequently throughout this cookbook. The Original Blend is an unusual assortment of sea salt, garlic, basil, rosemary, black pepper, and nutmeg that I often use on cuts of meat. The Citrus Seasoning Blend—similar to the original but with the inclusion of lemon peel—is a tasty blend that I often use with seafood. A.A. Borsari is available from upscale grocery stores nationwide or online. Other similar ingredient blends will work if you can't source Borsari.

SHORTENING: Whenever a recipe calls for shortening, I use Spectrum all-vegetable, non-hydrogenated shortening with zero trans fats.

SOY SAUCE VS. TAMARI: I often use tamari instead of soy sauce. Tamari is traditionally tied to the Japanese (versus the more common Chinese soy sauce). It is a thicker, less salty, fermented soy sauce that contains less wheat. Some brands of tamari are gluten-free.

VEGETABLE BOUILLON CUBE: Vegetable bouillon is called for in many of the recipes in this cookbook. I tested various brands. My favorite is Rapunzel with sea salt because I love the pop of its intense salty herb flavor. If you're sensitive to salt, Rapunzel also has a cube without salt.

CONVERSION CHARTS

The recipes in this cookbook use standard U.S. measures. The charts below offer equivalent measurements for grams and ounces. Liquid and dry measure equivalents, oven temperature conversions, and measurements for baking pans are also included.

BUTTER, CHEESE, AND SOLIDS CONVERSIONS

Measurement	Ounces	Grams
1 tablespoon = ⅛ stick	½ ounce	15 grams
2 tablespoons = ¼ stick	1 ounce	30 grams
4 tablespoons = ½ stick or ¼ cup	2 ounces	60 grams
8 tablespoons = 1 stick or ½ cup	4 ounces (¼ pound)	115 grams
16 tablespoons = 2 sticks or 1 cup	8 ounces (½ pound)	225 grams
32 tablespoons = 4 sticks or 2 cups	16 ounces (1 pound)	450 grams 500 grams = ½ kilogram

GRANULATED SUGAR CONVERSIONS

Measuring Spoons and Cups	Ounces	Grams
1 teaspoon	$\frac{1}{16}$ ounce	5 grams
1 tablespoon	½ ounce	15 grams
¼ cup (4 tablespoons)	1¾ ounces	60 grams
⅓ cup (5 tablespoons)	2¼ ounces	75 grams
½ cup	3½ ounces	100 grams
⅔ cup	4½ ounces	130 grams
¾ cup	5 ounces	150 grams
1 cup	7 ounces	200 grams
1½ cups	9½ ounces	300 grams
2 cups	13½ ounces	450 grams

FLOUR (UNSIFTED)

Measuring Spoons and Cups	Ounces	Grams
1 tablespoon	¼ ounce	8.75 grams
¼ cup (4 tablespoons)	1¼ ounces	35 grams
⅓ cup (5 tablespoons)	1½ ounces	45 grams
½ cup	2½ ounces	70 grams
⅔ cup	3¼ ounces	90 grams
¾ cup	3½ ounces	105 grams
1 cup	5 ounces	140 grams
1½ cups	7½ ounces	210 grams
2 cups	10 ounces	280 grams
3½ cups	16 ounces (1 pound)	490 grams

NOTE: 1 cup sifted flour = 1 cup unsifted flour minus 1½ tablespoons.

LIQUID AND DRY MEASUREMENT EQUIVALENTS

g = grams (dry measure), kg = kilograms, dL = deciliters, L = liters
The metric amounts represented here are the nearest equivalents.

A pinch = slightly less than ⅛ teaspoon
A dash = 3 drops
3 teaspoons = 1 tablespoon
2 tablespoons = 1 ounce = ¼ dL (liquid), 30 g (dry)
3 tablespoons = 1½ ounces
4 tablespoons = 2 ounces
8 tablespoons = ½ cup = 4 ounces = 1 dL
2 cups = 1 pint = ½ quart = 1 pound = ½ L (liquid), 450 g (dry)
4 cups = 32 ounces = 2 pints = 1 quart = 1 L
1 quart = about 1 L
4 quarts = 1 gallon = 3¾ L

OVEN TEMPERATURE CONVERSIONS

Fahrenheit	Celsius	Gas Mark
275° F	140° C	gas mark 1
300° F	150° C	gas mark 2
325° F	165° C	gas mark 3
350° F	180° C	gas mark 4
375° F	190° C	gas mark 5
400° F	200° C	gas mark 6
425° F	220° C	gas mark 7
450° F	230° C	gas mark 8
475° F	240° C	gas mark 9
500° F	260° C	gas mark 10

MEASUREMENTS FOR BAKING PANS

Baking Pans	Centimeters
8 x 8 x 2-inch baking pan	20 x 20 x 5 cm
9 x 9 x 2-inch baking pan	23 x 23 x 5 cm
11 x 7 x 2-inch baking pan	28 x 18 x 5 cm
13 x 9 x 2-inch baking pan	33 x 23 x 5 cm
15 x 10 x 2-inch baking pan	38 x 26 x 5 cm
9 x 5 x 3-inch loaf pan	23 x 13 x 6 cm
8 x 1½-inch cake pan	20 x 4 cm
9 x 1½-inch cake pan	23 x 4 cm
9-inch pie plate or baking dish	23 x 3 cm
10-inch pie plate or baking dish	25 x 5 cm
12½ x 17½ x 1-inch jelly roll pan	32 x 44 x 2.5 cm
2¾ x 1⅛-inch muffin pan (12 capacity)	7 x 3 cm

INDEX

A

all-purpose bread, 117-118

Almonds:
almond cookies, 227
almond lace cookies, 226
apricot, pistachio, and coconut granola, 142
chia-cherry muffins with almonds and millet, 156
gingered coconut and celery soup, 47
gingered turnip soup with coconut, 44
peach and cardamom coffee cake with almond butter streusel, 176-177
raspberry almond coffee cake with almond streusel, 173-174
toasted pesto crumbs, 149
wild rice salad with cherries and feta, 86

American-style meatloaf with pineapple glaze, 55

Apples:
lemon and ricotta apple cake, 203

Apricots:
apricot chia cake, 204
apricot, pistachio, and coconut granola, 142
apricot tomatoes with hearts of palm, shrimp, and feta, 73
chicken soup with couscous and apricots, 28
coconut curried cheese with mango chutney, 12
date and apricot muffins with walnuts and flaxseeds, 154
French-dressed apricot chicken wings, 15
savory-sweet apricot chicken, 61

Artichoke hearts:
lemon-marinated catfish with artichoke hearts and Kalamata olives, 72
roasted red pepper hummus dip with layered vegetables, feta, and olives, 5
vegetarian Mediterranean dip, 6

Arugula:
arugula, mango, and hearts of palm salad with salty lime dressing, 85
creamy shrimp and pasta with arugula pesto, 71
golden beet, arugula, pomegranate, and feta salad with blood orange dressing, 88

Asparagus:
asparagus and strawberry salad with grilled halloumi, 90-91
asparagus with crispy-fried shallots and brown butter bread crumbs, 93

Autumn spice:
apricot chia cake, 204
apricot, pistachio, and coconut granola, 142
autumn spice blend, 148
cranberry autumn spice bread, 111-112
date and autumn spice cake, 197
four-seed granola with molasses and cranberries, 143
pumpkin and millet muffins with autumn spice blend, 157

Avocado:
baked cod with toasted coconut and pineapple salsa, 74
coconut black bean soup with mango and avocado salsa, 41-42

B

Bacon:
egg noodles with creamed spinach and bacon, 60
fire-roasted tomato, eggplant, bacon, and bean casserole with poached eggs, 180-181
moist and delicious holiday turkey, 67-68
potato and corn chowder with bacon, 26

baked cod with toasted coconut and pineapple salsa, 74

Bananas:
banana upside-down pancakes, 168
blackened banana waffles, 171

basic white bread, 116

Basil:
coconut and roasted peanut ice cream with Thai basil, 230
Thai basil peanut pesto, 145
toasted pesto crumbs, 149

Beans, assorted:
beef, cheese, and black bean enchiladas, 54
cheesy eggplant, bean, and vegetable casserole, 77

chicken soup with couscous and apricots, 28

coconut black bean soup with mango and avocado salsa, 41-42

creamy coconut and cauliflower soup with tandoori spice, 27

fire-roasted seafood-style chili, 31

fire-roasted tomato, eggplant, bacon, and bean casserole with poached eggs, 180-181

green bean casserole soup, 45-46

ham and white bean soup, 29

herb-infused bean dip, 3

winter solstice soup, 48

Beef:
American-style meatloaf with pineapple glaze, 55

beef, cheese, and black bean enchiladas, 54

cast-iron New York strip steak, 52

creamed chipped beef with mushrooms, 56

moist and tender roast beef, 53

bittersweet chocolate cookies with sea salt, 222-223

blackened banana waffles, 171

Breads:
all-purpose bread, 117-118

basic white bread, 116

buttermilk bread, 119

cast-iron honey-glazed corn bread, 115

chia quinoa bread, 128-129

cranberry autumn spice bread, 111-112

dual seed tricolor quinoa bread, 123-124

grain and seed bread, 131-132

molasses-tinged pumpernickel raisin bread, 113-114

no-knead, all-purpose, country-style bread, 110

oatmeal bread, 130

pumpkin yeast bread, 120-121

seven whole grain bread, 126-127

spaghetti squash bread, 122

spelt bread with hemp seeds, 125

Brie:
new potatoes and shitake mushrooms with Brie, 102

Broccoli:
cheesy broccoli and mushroom dip, 10

creamy lemon penne pasta with broccoli, 78

sesame-roasted broccoli, 96

buttermilk bread, 119

Butternut squash:
buttery buttermilk Parmesan-stuffed potatoes, 101

gingered butternut squash soup with coconut, 37

C

Cabbage:
hearty cabbage and vegetable salad with celery seed dressing, 87

herbed cabbage and mushroom pie, 79-80

Cakes: see also coffee cake
apricot chia cake, 204

cardamom-infused cranberry cobbler cake, 200-201

chocolate-and-caramel-filled rolled cake, 208-209

chocolate-coconut-and-gingered-cranberry-cream-filled rolled cake, 212-213

chocolate cupcakes with chocolate pecan icing, 194-195

chocolate pomegranate wine cake, 196

clove-spiked red plum cake, 205

date and autumn spice cake, 197

fresh strawberry cake, 202

lemon and ricotta apple cake, 203

Mardi Gras sugar-glazed king pastry cake, 198-199

peaches-and-cream-filled rolled cake, 210-211

strawberry-and-cream-filled rolled cake, 206-207

Caramel:
caramel chocolate pie with salty pretzel crust, 214-215

caramel cream pie with salty pretzel crust, 216-217

chocolate-and-caramel-filled rolled cake, 208-209

cardamom-infused cranberry cobbler cake, 200-201

Casseroles:
cheesy eggplant, bean, and vegetable casserole, 77

company mushroom, sausage, and egg casserole, 182-183

fire-roasted tomato, eggplant, bacon, and bean casserole with poached eggs, 180-181

mushroom and spinach brunch casserole, 189-190

cast-iron honey-glazed corn bread, 115

cast-iron New York strip steak, 52

Cauliflower:
cauliflower and roasted red pepper quiche, 184-185
cauliflower soup with cheddar ciabatta toast, 24
chicken, vegetables, and brown rice pasta with red curry coconut sauce, 65-66
creamy coconut and cauliflower soup with tandoori spice, 27
curried cauliflower with toasted pecans, 94
curry cumin coconut cauliflower with prunes and peanuts, 98
hot cheddar and cauliflower dip, 9
marinated cauliflower, 97

Cheese tortellini:
vegetable chowder with cheese tortellini, 39

cheesy broccoli and mushroom dip, 10

cheesy eggplant, bean, and vegetable casserole, 77

Cherries:
cherry-and-cream-cheese-stuffed French toast, 172
chia-cherry muffins with almonds and millet, 156
coconut cherry muffins with pistachios, 160
wild rice salad with cherries and feta, 86

Chia seeds:
apricot chia cake, 204
chia-cherry muffins with almonds and millet, 156
chia quinoa bread, 128-129
oatmeal chia pancakes with ginger preserves, 165
quinoa chia pancakes, 164

Chicken:
chicken soup with couscous and apricots, 28
chicken, vegetables, and brown rice pasta with red curry coconut sauce, 65-66

curried cinnamon orange marmalade tomatoes with chicken and hearts of palm, 64
French-dressed apricot chicken wings, 15
lemon rosemary chicken wings, 11
maple Dijon glazed chicken, 63
savory-sweet apricot chicken, 61-62

Chocolate:
bittersweet chocolate cookies with sea salt, 222-223
caramel chocolate pie with salty pretzel crust, 214-215
chocolate-and-caramel-filled rolled cake, 208-209
chocolate-coconut-and-gingered-cranberry-cream-filled rolled cake, 212-213
chocolate, coconut, and peanut butter pie, 218
chocolate cupcakes with chocolate pecan icing, 194
chocolate fudge and pistachio nut cookies, 224
chocolate pomegranate wine cake, 196

Chowder:
potato and corn chowder with bacon, 26
vegetable chowder with cheese tortellini, 39

clove-spiked red plum cake, 205

Coconut:
apricot, pistachio, and coconut granola, 142
arugula, mango, and hearts of palm salad with salty lime dressing, 85
baked cod with toasted coconut and pineapple salsa, 74
chicken, vegetables, and brown rice pasta with red curry coconut sauce, 65-66
chocolate-coconut-and-gingered-cranberry-cream-filled rolled cake, 212-213
chocolate, coconut, and peanut butter pie, 218
coconut and mango lassi pancakes, 169
coconut and roasted peanut ice cream with Thai basil, 230
coconut black bean soup with mango and avocado salsa, 41-42
coconut cherry muffins with pistachios, 160
coconut cottage cheese pancakes, 162
coconut curried cheese with mango chutney, 12

coconut custard pie, 219
creamy coconut and cauliflower soup with
    tandoori spice, 27
curry cumin coconut cauliflower with
    prunes and peanuts, 98
gingered butternut squash soup with
    coconut, 37
gingered coconut and celery soup, 47
gingered turnip soup with coconut, 44
mango and coconut muffins, 155
pineapple and cardamom coffee cake with
    coconut macadamia streusel, 178-179
quinoa cheeseburgers with curried
    cucumber yogurt sauce, 75-76
shrimp and coconut soup with roasted corn
    and sweet potato, 33-34
Thai basil peanut pesto, 145
winter solstice soup, 48

Coffee cake:
peach and cardamom coffee cake with
    almond butter topping, 176-177
pineapple and cardamom coffee cake with
    coconut macadamia streusel, 178-179
pumpkin coffee cake with crunchy granola
    topping, 175
raspberry almond coffee cake with almond
    streusel, 173-174

Colman's deviled eggs with tarragon, 18

company mushroom, sausage, and egg
    casserole, 182-183

Cookies:
almond cookies, 227
almond lace cookies, 226
bittersweet chocolate cookies with sea salt,
    222-223
chocolate fudge and pistachio nut cookies,
    224
lemon crinkle cookies, 225

Corn:
cast-iron honey-glazed corn bread, 115
potato and corn chowder with bacon, 26
shrimp and coconut soup with roasted corn
    and sweet potato, 33-34

Cottage cheese:
coconut cottage cheese pancakes, 162
cottage cheese pancakes, 166

Couscous:
chicken soup with couscous and apricots, 28
poached eggs over couscous with a pop of
    harissa heat, 187-188

Crabmeat:
cucumber and crab soup, 35
Old Bay crab cakes, 69

Crawfish:
fire-roasted seafood-style chili, 31

cranberry autumn spice bread, 111-112

creamed chipped beef with mushrooms, 56

cream of turnip soup with pumpernickel
    croutons, 40

creamy coconut and cauliflower soup with
    tandoori spice, 27

creamy fire-roasted tomato soup, 25

creamy horseradish and chili sauce dip with
    shrimp, 4

creamy lemon penne pasta with broccoli, 78

creamy lobster soup, 32

creamy onion and red pepper cheese dip, 8

creamy shrimp and pasta with arugula pesto,
    71

creamy strawberry soup with Amaretto, 231

creamy wild mushroom soup with turmeric,
    38

Crepes:
simple buttermilk crepes, 144

Cucumbers:
cucumber and crab soup, 35
quinoa cheeseburgers with curried cucumber
    yogurt sauce, 75-76
roasted red pepper hummus dip with layered
    vegetables, feta, and olives, 5

Curry:
chicken, vegetables, and brown rice pasta
    with red curry coconut sauce, 65-66
coconut black bean soup with mango and
    avocado salsa, 41-42
coconut curried cheese with mango chutney,
    12
curried cauliflower with toasted pecans, 94

curried cinnamon orange marmalade tomatoes with chicken and hearts of palm, 64

curried pumpkin soup with mushrooms, 36

curry cumin coconut cauliflower with prunes and peanuts, 98

palak paneer, 81

quinoa cheeseburgers with curried cucumber yogurt sauce, 75-76

roasted curried potatoes, 105

shrimp and coconut soup with roasted corn and sweet potato, 33-34

tamari peanut sauce with toasted sesame and red curry, 147

winter solstice soup, 48

D

Dates:
date and apricot muffins with walnuts and flaxseeds, 154

date and autumn spice cake, 197

Deviled eggs:
Colman's deviled eggs with tarragon, 18

Dips:
cheesy broccoli and mushroom dip, 10

creamy horseradish and chili sauce dip with shrimp, 4

creamy onion and red pepper cheese dip, 8

herb-infused bean dip, 3

hot cheddar and cauliflower dip, 9

roasted red pepper hummus dip with layered vegetables, feta, and olives, 5

three-cheese and roasted vegetable dip, 7

vegetarian Mediterranean dip, 6

dual seed tricolor quinoa bread, 123-124

E

Egg dishes:
cauliflower and roasted red pepper quiche, 184-185

company mushroom, sausage, and egg casserole, 182-183

fire-roasted tomato, eggplant, bacon, and bean casserole with poached eggs, 180-181

mushroom and spinach brunch casserole, 189-190

poached eggs over couscous with a pop of harissa heat, 187-188

scrambled eggs with thyme, 186

egg noodles with creamed spinach and bacon, 60

Eggplant:
cheesy eggplant, bean, and vegetable casserole, 77

fire-roasted tomato, eggplant, bacon, and bean casserole with poached eggs, 180-181

Enchiladas:
beef, cheese, and black bean enchiladas, 54

F

fire-roasted seafood-style chili, 31

fire roasted tomato, eggplant, bacon, and bean casserole with poached eggs, 180-181

Fish:
baked cod with toasted coconut and pineapple salsa, 74

herbed trout with fried carrots, 70

lemon-marinated catfish with artichoke hearts and Kalamata olives, 72

Flaxseeds:
coconut cherry muffins with pistachios, 160

date and apricot muffins with walnuts and flaxseeds, 154

dual seed tricolor quinoa bread, 123-124

grain and seed bread, 131-132

pumpkin coffee cake with crunchy granola topping, 175

quinoa muffins with flaxseed and sunflower seeds, 159

four-seed granola with molasses and cranberries, 143

French-dressed apricot chicken wings, 15

French toast:
cherry-and-cream-cheese-stuffed French toast, 172

fresh strawberry cake, 202

frozen margarita martinis with salty pretzel crust, 228-229

G

Ginger:

chocolate-coconut-and-gingered-cranberry-
cream-filled rolled cake, 212-213

gingered butternut squash soup with
coconut, 37

gingered coconut and celery soup, 47

gingered cranberry sauce, 150

gingered mango pancakes, 161

gingered tomatoes with cinnamon, 100

gingered turnip soup with coconut, 44

oatmeal chia pancakes with ginger preserves,
165

palak paneer, 81

golden beet, arugula, pomegranate, and feta
salad with blood orange dressing, 88

grain and seed bread, 131-132

Granola:

apricot, pistachio, and coconut granola, 142

four-seed granola with molasses and
cranberries, 143

pumpkin coffee cake with crunchy granola
topping, 175

Green beans:
green bean casserole soup, 45-46

H

Ham:
ham and white bean soup, 29

Hearts of palm:

apricot tomatoes with hearts of palm,
shrimp, and feta, 73

arugula, mango, and hearts of palm salad
with salty lime dressing, 85

hearty cabbage and vegetable salad with celery
seed dressing, 87

Herbs:

herbed cabbage and mushroom pie, 79-80

herbed trout with fried carrots, 70

herb garlic butter, 146

herb-infused bean dip, 3

heirloom tomato and mozzarella salad with
toasted pesto crumbs, 89

honey-buttered peppered turnips with sweet
peas, 99

hot cheddar and cauliflower dip, 9

Hummus:

roasted red pepper hummus dip with layered
vegetables, feta, and olives, 5

vegetarian Mediterranean dip, 6

I

Ice cream:

coconut and roasted peanut ice cream with
Thai basil, 230

K

Kalamata olives:

lemon-marinated catfish with artichoke
hearts and Kalamata olives, 72

poached eggs over couscous with a pop of
harissa heat, 187-188

roasted red pepper hummus dip with layered
vegetables, feta, and olives, 5

vegetarian Mediterranean dip, 6

L

Lamb:

leg of lamb roast stuffed with spinach, feta,
and pine nuts, 57-58

Lasagna:
wild porcini mushroom lasagna, 82

Lassi:
coconut and mango lassi pancakes, 169

Lemon:

creamy lemon penne pasta with broccoli, 78

lemon and ricotta apple cake, 208

lemon crinkle cookies, 225

lemon-marinated catfish with artichoke
hearts and Kalamata olives, 72

lemon rosemary chicken wings, 11

Lobster:

creamy lobster soup, 32

New England-like lobster pies, 16

M

Macadamia nuts:

baked cod with toasted coconut and
pineapple salsa, 74

pineapple and cardamom coffee cake with
coconut macadamia streusel, 178-179

Mango:

arugula, mango, and hearts of palm salad
with salty lime dressing, 85

coconut and mango lassi pancakes, 169

coconut black bean soup with mango and avocado salsa, 41-42

coconut curried cheese with mango chutney, 12

gingered mango pancakes, 161

mango and coconut muffins, 155

mango waffles, 170

maple Dijon glazed chicken, 63

Mardi Gras sugar-glazed king pastry cake, 198-199

marinated cauliflower, 97

Meatloaf:

    American-style meatloaf with pineapple glaze, 55

Millet:

    chia-cherry muffins with almonds and millet, 156

    pumpkin and millet muffins with autumn spice blend, 157-158

moist and delicious holiday turkey, 67-68

molasses-tinged pumpernickel raisin bread, 113-114

Muffins:

    chia-cherry muffins with almonds and millet, 156

    coconut cherry muffins with pistachios, 160

    date and apricot muffins with walnuts and flaxseeds, 154

    mango and coconut muffins, 155

    pumpkin and millet muffins with autumn spice blend, 157-158

    quinoa muffins with flaxseed and sunflower seeds, 159

Mushrooms:

    chessy broccoli and mushroom dip, 10

    chicken, vegetables, and brown rice pasta with red curry coconut sauce, 65-66

    company mushroom, sausage, and egg casserole, 182-183

    creamed chipped beef with mushrooms, 56

    creamy lobster soup, 32

    creamy wild mushroom soup with turmeric, 38

    curried pumpkin soup with mushroms, 36

    green bean casserole soup, 45-46

    herbed cabbage and mushroom pie, 79-80

    mushroom and spinach brunch casserole, 189-190

    mushroom soup with spinach tortellini, 43

    new potatoes with shitake mushrooms and Brie, 102

    puff pastry with creamy mushroom filling, 13-14

    vegetable chowder with cheese tortellini, 39

    wild porcini mushroom lasagna, 82

N

New England-like lobster pies, 16

new potatoes with shitake mushrooms and Brie, 102

no-knead, all-purpose, country-style bread, 110

Nuts, *see specific nuts*

O

oatmeal bread, 130

oatmeal chia pancakes with ginger preserves, 165

Old Bay crab cakes, 69

P

palak paneer, 81

Pancakes:

    banana upside-down pancakes, 168

    coconut and mango lassi pancakes, 169

    coconut cottage cheese pancakes, 162

    cottage cheese pancakes, 166

    gingered mango pancakes, 161

    oatmeal chia pancakes with ginger preserves, 165

    pineapple upside-down pancakes, 167

    quinoa chia pancakes, 164

    raspberry pancakes, 163

Parsnips:

    savory-sweet parsnip and sweet potato soup, 30

Pasta:

    chicken, vegetables, and brown rice pasta with red curry coconut sauce, 65-66

    creamy lemon penne pasta with broccoli, 78

    creamy shrimp and pasta with arugula pesto, 71

egg noodles with creamed spinach and
bacon, 60
wild porcini mushroom lasagna, 82

see also tortellini

Peaches:
peach and cardamom coffee cake with
almond butter streusel, 176-177
peaches-and-cream-filled rolled cake, 210-
211

Peanut butter:
chicken, vegetables, and brown rice pasta
with red curry coconut sauce, 65-66
chocolate, coconut, and peanut butter pie,
218
coconut black bean soup with mango and
avocado salsa, 41-42
creamy coconut and cauliflower soup with
tandoori spice, 27
tamari peanut sauce with toasted sesame and
red curry, 147

Peanuts:
coconut and roasted peanut ice cream with
Thai basil, 230
curry cumin coconut cauliflower with
prunes and peanuts, 98
Thai basil peanut pesto, 145

Pecans:
chocolate cupcakes with chocolate pecan
icing, 194-195
coconut curried cheese with mango chutney,
12
curried cauliflower with toasted pecans, 94
Mardi Gras sugar-glazed king pastry cake,
198-199

Pesto:
creamy shrimp and pasta with arugula pesto,
71
heirloom tomato and mozzarella salad with
toasted pesto crumbs, 89
Thai basil peanut pesto, 145
toasted pesto crumbs, 149

Phyllo shells:
New England-like lobster pies, 16

Pies:
caramel chocolate pie with salty pretzel
crust, 214-215

caramel cream pie with salty pretzel crust,
216-217
chocolate, coconut, and peanut butter pie,
218
coconut custard pie, 219
herbed cabbage and mushroom pie, 79-80
New England-like lobster pies, 16
rhubarb pie, 220-221

Pineapple:
American-style meatloaf with pineapple
glaze, 55
baked cod with toasted coconut and
pineapple salsa, 74
pineapple and cardamom coffee cake with
coconut macadamia streusel, 178-179
pineapple rum whipped cream, 139
pineapple upside-down pancakes, 167

Pine nuts:
leg of lamb roast stuffed with spinach, feta,
and pine nuts, 57-58

Pistachios:
apricot, pistachio, and coconut granola, 142
chocolate fudge and pistachio nut cookies,
224
coconut cherry muffins with pistachios, 160

Pizza:
thick crust pizza, 133-134
thin crust pizza, 135

Plums:
clove-spiked red plum cake, 205

Pomegranate:
chocolate pomegranate wine cake, 196
golden beet, arugula, pomegranate, and feta
salad with blood orange dressing, 88

Pork:
pork tenderloin with roasted coffee and
allspice, 59

Potatoes, white:
buttery buttermilk Parmesan-stuffed
potatoes, 101
cream of turnip soup with pumpernickel
croutons, 40
new potatoes with shitake mushrooms and
Brie, 102
potato and corn chowder with bacon, 26
roasted curried potatoes, 105
roasted potatoes with minted garlic, 103

simple creamy potatoes, 104

Puff pastry:
    puff pastry with creamy mushroom filling, 13-14
    spinach-stuffed puff pastry, 95

Pumpernickel:
    cream of turnip soup with pumpernickel croutons, 40
    molasses-tinged pumpernickel raisin bread, 113-114

Pumpkin:
    curried pumpkin soup with mushrooms, 36
    pumpkin and millet muffins with autumn spice blend, 157-158
    pumpkin coffee cake with crunchy granola topping, 175
    pumpkin yeast bread, 120-121

Q

Quiche:
    cauliflower and roasted red pepper quiche, 184-185

Quinoa:
    chia quinoa bread, 128-129
    dual seed tricolor quinoa bread, 123-124
    grain and seed bread, 131-132
    quinoa cheeseburgers with curried cucumber yogurt sauce, 75-76
    quinoa chia pancakes, 164
    quinoa muffins with flaxseed and sunflower seeds, 159

quintessential Caesar salad, 92

R

Raspberries:
    raspberry almond coffee cake with almond streusel, 173-174
    raspberry almond whipped cream, 140
    raspberry pancakes, 163

Rhubarb:
    rhubarb pie, 220-221

roasted curried potatoes, 105

roasted potatoes with minted garlic, 103

roasted red pepper hummus dip with layered vegetables, feta, and olives, 5

S

Salads:
    arugula, mango, and hearts of palm salad with salty lime dressing, 85
    asparagus and strawberry salad with grilled halloumi, 90-91
    golden beet, arugula, pomegranate, and feta salad with blood orange dressing, 88
    hearty cabbage and vegetable salad with celery seed dressing, 87
    heirloom tomato and mozzarella salad with toasted pesto crumbs, 89
    quintessential Caesar salad, 92
    wild rice salad with cherries and feta, 86

Salsa:
    baked cod with toasted coconut and pineapple salsa, 74
    coconut black bean soup with mango and avocado salsa, 41-42

Sausage:
    company mushroom, sausage, and egg casserole, 182-183

savory-sweet apricot chicken, 61-62

savory-sweet parsnip and sweet potato soup, 30

scrambled eggs with thyme, 186

Seafood: crabmeat, crawfish, fish, lobster, shrimp:
    apricot tomatoes with hearts of palm, shrimp, and feta, 73
    baked cod with toasted coconut and pineapple salsa, 74
    creamy lobster soup, 32
    creamy shrimp and pasta with arugula pesto, 71
    cucumber and crab soup, 35
    fire-roasted seafood-style chili, 31
    herbed trout with fried carrots, 70
    lemon-marinated catfish with artichoke hearts and Kalamata olives, 72
    New England-like lobster pies, 16
    Old Bay crab cakes, 69
    shrimp and coconut soup with roasted corn and sweet potato, 33-34
    see also crabmeat, crawfish, fish, lobster, shrimp

sesame-roasted broccoli, 96

seven whole grain bread, 126-127

Shrimp:
    apricot tomatoes with hearts of palm,
        shrimp, and feta, 73
    creamy horseradish and chili sauce dip with
        shrimp, 4
    creamy shrimp and pasta with arugula pesto,
        71
    fire-roasted seafood-style chili, 31
    shrimp and coconut soup with roasted corn
        and sweet potato, 33-34

simple buttermilk crepes, 144

simple creamy potatoes, 104

Soups:
    cauliflower soup with cheddar ciabatta toast,
        24
    chicken soup with couscous and apricots, 28
    coconut black bean soup with mango and
        avocado salsa, 41-42
    cream of turnip soup with pumpernickel
        croutons, 40
    creamy coconut and cauliflower soup with
        tandoori spice, 27
    creamy fire-roasted tomato soup, 25
    creamy lobster soup, 32
    creamy strawberry soup with Amaretto, 231
    creamy wild mushroom soup with turmeric,
        38
    cucumber and crab soup, 35
    curried pumpkin soup with mushrooms, 36
    fire-roasted seafood-style chili, 31
    gingered butternut squash soup with
        coconut, 37
    gingered coconut and celery soup, 47
    gingered turnip soup with coconut, 44
    green bean casserole soup, 45-46
    ham and white bean soup, 29
    mushroom soup with spinach tortellini, 43
    potato and corn chowder with bacon, 26
    savory-sweet parsnip and sweet potato soup,
        30
    shrimp and coconut soup with roasted corn
        and sweet potato, 33-34
    vegetable chowder with cheese tortellini, 39
    winter solstice soup, 48
    see also chowders

Spaghetti squash:
    spaghetti squash bread, 122
    three-cheese spaghetti squash fritters, 19-20

spelt bread with hemp seeds, 125

Spinach:
    egg noodles with creamed spinach and
        bacon, 60
    fire-roasted tomato, eggplant, bacon, and
        bean casserole with poached eggs, 180-
        181
    leg of lamb roast stuffed with spinach, feta,
        and pine nuts, 57-58
    mushroom and spinach brunch casserole,
        189-190
    mushroom soup with spinach tortellini, 43
    palak paneer, 81
    spinach Parmesan bites, 17
    spinach-stuffed puff pastry, 95
    vegetarian Mediterranean dip, 6

Squash, see also specific squash:
    gingered butternut squash soup with
        coconut, 37
    spaghetti squash bread, 122
    three-cheese spaghetti squash fritters, 19-20

Steak:
    cast-iron New York strip steak, 52

Strawberries:
    asparagus and strawberry salad with grilled
        halloumi, 90-91
    creamy strawberry soup with Amaretto, 231
    fresh strawberry cake, 202
    strawberry Amaretto whipped cream, 141
    strawberry-and-cream-filled rolled cake,
        206-207

Sunflower seeds:
    apricot, pistachio, and coconut granola, 142
    four-seed granola with molasses and
        cranberries, 143
    golden beet, arugula, pomegranate, and feta
        salad with blood orange dressing, 88
    hearty cabbage and vegetable salad with
        celery seed dressing, 87
    quinoa muffins with flaxseed and sunflower
        seeds, 159

Sweet potatoes:
    creamy coconut and cauliflower soup with
        tandoori spice, 27
    savory-sweet parsnip and sweet potato soup,
        30
    shrimp and coconut soup with roasted corn
        and sweet potato, 33-34

T

tamari peanut sauce with toasted sesame and red curry, 147

Thai basil peanut pesto, 145

thick crust pizza, 133-134

thin crust pizza, 135

three-cheese and roasted vegetable dip, 7

three-cheese spaghetti squash fritters, 19-20

toasted pesto crumbs, 149

Tomatoes:
    apricot tomatoes with hearts of palm, shrimp, and feta, 73
    cheesy eggplant, bean, and vegetable casserole, 77
    creamy coconut and cauliflower soup with tandoori spice, 27
    creamy fire-roasted tomato soup, 25
    curried cinnamon orange marmalade tomatoes with chicken and hearts of palm, 64
    fire-roasted seafood-style chili, 31
    fire-roasted tomato, eggplant, bacon, and bean casserole with poached eggs, 180-181
    gingered tomatoes with cinnamon, 100
    heirloom tomato and mozzarella salad with toasted pesto crumbs, 89
    mushroom soup with spinach tortellini, 43
    savory-sweet apricot chicken, 61-62
    shrimp and coconut soup with roasted corn and sweet potato, 33-34
    winter solstice soup, 48

Tomatoes, sun-dried:
    leg of lamb roast stuffed with spinach, feta, and pine nuts, 57-58
    roasted red pepper hummus dip with layered vegetables, feta, and olives, 5

Tortellini:
    mushroom soup with spinach tortellini, 43
    vegetable chowder with cheese tortellini, 39

Trout:
    herbed trout with fried carrots, 70

Turkey:
    moist and delicious holiday turkey, 67-68

Turnips:
    cream of turnip soup with pumpernickel croutons, 40
    gingered turnip soup with coconut, 44
    honey-buttered peppered turnips and sweet peas, 99

V

vegetable chowder with cheese tortellini, 39

vegetarian Mediterranean dip, 6

W

Waffles:
    blackened banana waffles, 171
    mango waffles, 170

Walnuts:
    date and apricot muffins with walnuts and flaxseeds, 154

wild porcini mushroom lasagna, 82

Wild rice:
    creamy coconut and cauliflower soup with tandoori spice, 27
    wild rice salad with cherries and feta, 86

winter solstice soup, 48

ABOUT THE AUTHOR

Kerry Dunnington was born in the suburbs of Baltimore, Maryland, where she lived with her parents and five siblings. At an early age, she developed her palate for fresh and delicious-tasting meals prepared from scratch by her mother—a self-taught home cook. Kerry has published three cookbooks, including *Tasting the Seasons* and *This Book Cooks,* which have won nine national book awards. Owner of Kerry Dunnington Catering since 1992, Kerry has also been a popular food columnist, culinary consultant, food judge, and recipe developer for more than three decades. She makes frequent appearances at farmers' markets around Maryland, where she collaborates with farmers, food vendors, and artisans to showcase their fresh bounty with recipes from her cookbooks. Kerry's home—and the kitchen where she creates the trademark dishes enjoyed by her husband, Nick, and their Norwich terrier, Caramel—is in a century-old co-op in Baltimore's historic Tuscany-Canterbury neighborhood.

NOTES

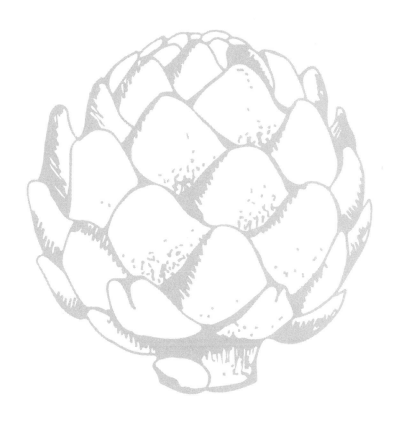